MW00581997

SACRED KNOWLEDGE

Sacred Knowledge

PSYCHEDELICS AND RELIGIOUS EXPERIENCES

William A. Richards

Foreword by G. William Barnard

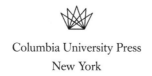

Columbia University Press

New York

Columbia University Press
Publishers Since 1893
New York   Chichester, West Sussex
cup.columbia.edu

Library of Congress Cataloging-in-Publication Data

Richards, William A., 1940–
    Sacred knowledge : psychedelics and religious experiences / William A. Richards
        pages cm
    Includes bibliographical references and index.
    ISBN 978-0-231-17406-0 (cloth : alk. paper) – ISBN 978-0-231-54091-9 (e-book)
    1. Hallucinogenic drugs and religious experience.   I. Title.

BL65.D7R53   2015
204'.2–dc23   2015014533

∞

Columbia University Press books are printed on permanent and durable acid-free paper.
This book is printed on paper with recycled content.
Printed in the United States of America

Cover design: Face-Out Studio
Cover art: Edna Kurtz Emmet/ednakurtzemmet.com

To my sons, Daniel and Brian

One must say that revelatory experiences are universally human. Religions are based on something that is given to man wherever he lives, namely, revelation, a particular kind of experience which always implies saving powers. You can never separate revelation and salvation. God has not left Himself unwitnessed.

–Paul Tillich (1886–1965), *The Future of Religions*

Man is always more than he knows about himself.

–Karl Jaspers (1883–1969), *The Perennial Scope of Philosophy*

Religiously conceived, the human opportunity is to transform flashes of illumination into abiding light.

–Huston Smith (b. 1919), *Cleansing the Doors of Perception*

CONTENTS

FOREWORD

G. WILLIAM BARNARD

The book that you are about to read is a treasure.

But before I describe what awaits you within this text, I want to say a few words about the book's author, Bill Richards, a crucially important figure in the tradition of psychedelic researchers and therapists.

I vividly remember the first time that I had the good fortune to meet Dr. Richards, when he came to visit me in Dallas a few years ago on his way to south Texas. When I went to pick him up at the DFW airport, I knew the bare basics about his background, but I didn't know what he looked like. So, as I was scanning the people who were streaming into the baggage claim area to pick up their luggage, I wondered how I would ever recognize him.

I shouldn't have worried. It was immediately clear to me: "that's him," the tall man with a shock of white hair and glasses who was standing there with a huge elfin grin on his face and (almost literal) twinkles in his eyes, the man who clearly was enjoying every moment of that crowded, noisy baggage claim area.

I immediately knew that we were going to hit it off.

I wasn't mistaken.

Dr. Richards is that rare example of a scientifically rigorous, tremendously learned intellectual who, nonetheless, is genuinely lit up from within. He is someone who, instead of just talking about sacred knowledge, psychedelics, and religious experiences, has clearly taken his own advice and has somehow managed to become, if I may be so bold, a shining example of a living mystic, a walking, talking, genuine, real-deal sage–all the while remaining extremely down-to-earth, witty, and warm.

As you begin to read *Sacred Knowledge*, I am sure that it will quickly become clear that the author is someone who has mulled over a whole host of complex and profound issues for quite a long time, and has something to say that he believes is deeply worthwhile. This book is not only extremely timely and relevant; it also addresses, with seemingly effortless ease, many of the subtler metaphysical implications of psychedelics–that is, it doesn't just deal with the enormous therapeutic potential of these substances, but also their tremendous spiritual potential as well. These aren't topics that are easy to address, but with his lucid prose, his gentle, self-effacing humor, and his distinctive voice (genial yet learned, heartfelt yet straightforward), Dr. Richards makes articulating such difficult topics look easy.

As an elder of the psychedelic movement, Dr. Richards offers his readers something precious: his own decades-long, deeply hands-on experience with psychedelic research. He was there during the early 1960s, a time in which he, along with numerous friends and colleagues, first began (with enormous hope and optimism) to research the potential psychological and spiritual benefits of psychedelics. (Dr. Richards was a close friend with Walter Pahnke, the lead researcher for the famous "Good Friday Experiment" that took place on April 20, 1962, in Boston University's Marsh Chapel, when twenty students from the Andover-Newton Theological School took part in a double-blind study that was designed to ascertain whether psilocybin could reliably induce mystical experiences.) Dr. Richards was also there in 1977, when (as he puts it) he had the "dubious distinction" of acting as the last researcher and clinician to administer psilocybin to a patient at the Maryland Psychiatric Research Center–the only institution at that time in the United States that was legally allowed to conduct research on psychedelic substances. Then, in 1999, when the tide shifted toward a more sane and nuanced response to psychedelic substances, Dr. Richards was at the forefront of the reinitiation of responsible, careful research on psychedelics, research that began at the Johns Hopkins School of Medicine and that eventually expanded to other centers of study in North America and Europe and that continues on to this day.

Throughout this book, Dr. Richards draws upon this enormous wealth of experience as he (rather adroitly) switches between, on the one hand, skillfully discussing the high points of decades of scientific research on psychedelics and, on the other hand, discussing with subtlety and care a wide range of profound religious and metaphysical topics. I will admit that, for myself at least, it is refreshing to see, in our current intellectual climate, which often values disengagement, skepticism, and irony, how Dr. Richards is willing to speak passionately and clearly from his heart about subjects that many (if not most) academics shy away from, such as healing, finding meaning, and spiritual awakening.

These crucially significant topics are addressed from three distinct perspectives. First, Dr. Richards speaks from his decades of clinical work, as someone who has legally and openly, for over twenty-five years, utilized and researched the effects of a variety of psychedelics within a therapeutic context and is therefore able to include numerous riveting first-person accounts of his patients' experiences with these substances and the subsequent transformative effects on their lives. Second, Dr. Richards writes out of his (again) decades-long immersion in, and lively engagement with, the religious and philosophical literature that focuses on the study of mysticism and other "nonordinary" states of consciousness. Third, Dr. Richards offers us a few judiciously chosen and clearly described accounts of his own experiences with psychedelics. In a straightforward, completely nonironic (but not in any way naïve) way, he is willing to make the bold and perhaps (at least to many people) rather startling claim that psychedelic substances, if taken in the proper context and with a specific mind-set or intentionality, can and do reliably catalyze genuine mystical and visionary experiences.

I think that this deeply courageous claim needs to be taken seriously. Speaking personally, as someone who has dedicated his entire professional career to a careful examination of the psychological and philosophical implications of mystical experiences and other "nonordinary" states of consciousness, and as someone who has spent numerous years studying the Santo Daime tradition, a religion that centers on the sacramental ingestion of the psychedelic substance ayahuasca, I am persuaded that powerful psychedelic experiences are far from being pathological hallucinatory misfirings of our brain circuitry. They are instead, at least potentially, genuine encounters with not only typically hidden strata of our psyche, but also levels of reality that deserve, if anything does, to be called "sacred." As a scholar of mysticism, what is so striking to me about this text is that Dr. Richards, after having clearly immersed himself in the literature that surrounds this rather arcane (yet important) topic, is able to demonstrate, thoroughly and compellingly, the striking correspondence between the key qualities of classical mystical states of awareness and the states of conscious-ness that arise when, for example, a volunteer in one of his research studies is given a powerful dose of psilocybin. (Perhaps equally, if not more, impressive are the accounts of the transformative effects of such experiences in the daily lives of those who took part in these studies.)

Again, speaking personally, it is my hope that this book will help to dispel the decades of deeply distorted misinformation (if not outright falsehoods) that has characterized our nation's decades-long repressive attack on psychedelics. Here, at last, are words of moderation, words of clarity, words of sanity, on this highly sensationalized topic. As this text so clearly notes, psychedelics should in no way be confused with highly addictive, often toxic drugs, such as heroin, cocaine, metham-phetamines (and yes, let's say it openly, alcohol and nicotine). Unlike these often deeply destructive drugs, the substances that Dr. Richards focuses on in this text (for example, LSD, mescaline, psilocybin, and DMT) are nonaddictive and nontoxic. Furthermore, as this text so vividly shows, if taken or administered responsibly within a skilled psychotherapeutic or religious context, these substances also have the potential to have tremendous therapeutic, as well as spiritual, value.

Dr. Richards is by no means advocating psychedelics as some sort of panacea. He is keenly aware of the risks that can arise from the irresponsible, hedonistic misuse of these powerful substances. None-theless, Dr. Richards is also cognizant of the thousands of careful stud-ies that took place in over a decade of intensive clinical and scientific research in the late 1950s, 1960s, and early 1970s that demonstrated, time and time again, that these substances have clear psychotherapeutic and medical potential (the treatment of alcoholism was particularly promising). Dr. Richards also knows, from his rich experience as a clinician, the enormous potential rewards that can arise with the carefully monitored use of these substances. The book's description of the psychotherapeutic and spiritual breakthroughs of his research subjects and clinical patients is perhaps one of the highlights of the text.

In this book, Dr. Richards devotes significant attention to the implications of some of the most crucial and startling findings of this research. If, as seems to be the case, the experiences that are catalyzed by these substances are indistinguishable from the mystical accounts that fill the religious literature of every major religious tradition, then scientists and scholars have been given a rare and precious opportunity: mystical experiences, which typically are extremely ephemeral and unpredictable, can actually be catalyzed in a fairly reliable and replicable way with the correct use of psychedelic substances (that is, if carefully prepared volunteers, with worthwhile goals and in a comfortable and uplifting setting, are given the right dosage). The crucial implications of this opportunity for the study of mysticism cannot be understated: these exalted states of consciousness, once so rare and difficult to study, can now be fairly reliably accessed, and hence can be carefully and respectfully investigated by scholars, scientists, clinicians, and religious professionals within safe and responsible settings.

Dr. Richards also does not shy away from the implications of this research for fundamental questions about the nature of selfhood and even about the nature of reality itself. Dr. Richards, with his calm and lucid prose, approaches these topics in a subtle and yet systematic manner. Page by page he unfolds his vision of the wondrous depths of the psyche and the equally wondrous underlying beauty of this world–a vision that, in his case, is not simply lofty yet unsubstantiated metaphysical speculation, but rather buttressed by the compelling and detailed accounts of the experiences and insights of his patients and research volunteers (as well as by narratives of his own generously offered and lucidly written experiences).

This text also offers calm and sober advice on how to deal with psychosomatic distress while taking psychedelic substances; how (when taking these substances) to maximize the potential for safely receiving a psychologically and spiritually transformative mystical experience; how to best integrate these profound experiences into one's daily life; how these substances can potentially give meaning to both daily life and the experience of dying; how psychedelics can help survivors to cope with the grief associated with the death of a loved one; and finally, the rather astonishing potential of these substances to deal with various severe addictions as well as clinical depression. (The recent study at Johns Hopkins that found an 80 percent abstinence rate from nicotine addiction after only three psilocybin treatments combined with cognitive-behavioral therapy is, at least to me, especially intriguing.) Dr. Richards is even willing, in his incurably optimistic way, to offer several thoughtful and intriguing musings on the potential of these substances for increased creativity in the arts, sciences, and even religious life.

For any reader interested in the therapeutic and mystical implications of psychedelics, this book will be both eye-opening and richly rewarding. Enjoy!

PREFACE

One Discovery of Transcendence

When my own first intense encounter with mystical consciousness occurred, I was a twenty-three-year-old graduate student of theology and psychiatry. Studying at the University of Göttingen in Germany, formally known as the Georg-August Universität, I had volunteered to participate in a research project with a drug I had never heard about called psilocybin. Synthesized and distributed to psychiatric researchers and clinicians by the Sandoz Pharmaceutical Company in Switzerland, this new drug was the primary psychoactive substance in the *psilocybe* genus of mushrooms that indigenous peoples had called "magic" or "sacred" and appear to have used in their religious practices for at least three thousand years and perhaps since as long ago as 5000 BCE. On this date in the modern world, December 4, 1963, however, the dark ages of psychedelic research still prevailed and, in the context of Western psychopharmacological investigations, drugs like psilocybin usually were administered without preparation or guidance.

At the time, it was hoped that the radically different, sometimes disorganized or psychotic states of consciousness that often ensued, fortunately temporary in duration, would advance our understanding of schizophrenia and similar states of mind. Hanscarl Leuner, the professor of psychiatry conducting the investigations in the

Nervenklinik in Göttingen, just had published a scientific monograph on his observations titled *Die experimentelle Psychose* (The Experimental Psychoses). In those days psychedelic drugs were freely available to qualified researchers in Europe and in the United States, sent through the mail. Psilocybin was marketed as Indocybin. The distribution of LSD, known as Delysid, as stated in a 1964 Sandoz pamphlet, was simply "restricted to psychiatrists for use in mental hospitals and psychiatric clinics."

Not only did I know nothing about psilocybin, LSD, or mescaline, I had not yet even heard the term "psychedelic," though it had been coined seven years earlier by Humphrey Osmond, a British psychiatrist, in a letter to Aldous Huxley. However, two of my new friends reported to me that they had volunteered for an interesting research project in the nearby psychiatric clinic that entailed receiving an experimental drug. Its name was hard to remember, but it was reputed to provide some insights into early childhood. One friend had experienced himself sitting in his father's lap and, since his father had been killed in World War II, this was profoundly comforting and meaningful to him. The other had seen visionary imagery of Nazi SS soldiers marching in the streets that he called "a hallucination." I was intrigued and, being curious about the psychodynamic processes in my early childhood and having never seen a "real hallucination," decided to walk over to the clinic and inquire whether I also could qualify as a participant in the research project. I viewed my own mind as a psychological laboratory in those days, took myself much too seriously, and sometimes went without breakfast to write down my dreams in the morning. Somewhat pompously, I called this discipline "collecting my phenomenological data." (I was fond of big words then! In retrospect I realize that a healthy breakfast might have done me much more good.)

I found that I was permitted to apply and submitted myself to a cursory medical screening. I remember being asked if I got drunk very often (I didn't). Then, informed I was acceptable, I was led to a rather dim and drab basement room, just large enough for a cot, an end table, and a chair. I met Gerhard Baer, a pleasant psychiatric resident about my age who wore a spiffy white coat with a stethoscope. After a brief chat, he gave me an injection of a derivative of psilocybin in liquid form. Though periodically observed during the next three to four hours, basically I then was left alone. Drawing on the piety of my Methodist childhood, I silently affirmed trust that God would be with me should any difficult childhood memories emerge.

To my utter amazement, I soon discovered in my visual field the emergence of an exquisitely beautiful, multidimensional network of intricate, neon-like geometric patterns, drawing my attention ever more deeply within. I could see this display with open eyes, but found that when I closed my eyes it was even more vivid and sharply focused. I recognized life within the undulating designs and began to feel as though I somehow could enter into the energy flowing within them. Soon, I felt immersed in incredibly detailed imagery best described as Islamic architecture and Arabic script, about which I knew nothing. Then (forgive the poetic license), I seemed to fully become the multidimensional patterns or to lose my usual identity within them as the eternal brilliance of mystical consciousness manifested itself. Suddenly this consciousness was experienced as outside of time, a pinnacle from which history could be viewed. My awareness was flooded with love, beauty, and peace beyond anything I ever had known or wildly imagined to be possible. "Awe," "Glory," and "Gratitude" were the only words that remained relevant.

For a few moments "back on earth," as garbage men emptied the clinic's metal cans in the alley outside the room's narrow window, I faintly registered tinkling temple bells. There were also a few minutes when Gerhard entered the room and asked me to sit on the edge of the cot with my legs crossed so he could test my knee reflexes. I recall complying with his request, silently holding my arms outstretched with open palms. Intently, he struck my patellar tendons with his little hammer and jotted down his findings while I felt what I later called "compassion for the infancy of science." I was aware that the researchers appeared to have no idea of what really was happening in my inner experiential world, of its unspeakable beauty or of its potential importance for all of us.

When left alone again, immersed in awe, eventually my ego or everyday personality reconstituted itself enough to fear that I somehow might forget the utterly convincing reality of this magnificent state of consciousness. Tentatively, I established again that my body indeed could move. Then, I stretched out my right arm to grasp a piece of blue paper on the end table beside me, picked up a pencil, and wrote, "Realität ist. Es ist vielleicht nicht wichtig was man darüber denkt!" (Reality is. It is perhaps not important what one thinks about it!) I underlined the first "ist" three times.

After returning to normative consciousness about four hours after the injection and futilely trying to describe something of my experience to Gerhard, I walked slowly and thoughtfully back to my dormitory room in the Uhlhorn Studienkonvikt, a short distance away from the clinic. I climbed to the fourth floor, softly opened and closed the door of my room, and immediately lay prostrate on the wide, rough, highly waxed floorboards like a monk before an altar, speechless with reverence and gratitude. I was thankful for privacy, well aware that if others were observing me they might view my behavior as rather strange, if not downright crazy. Intuitively I felt that all was well and did not want well-meaning friends to worry about me.

A few days later, still in awe over what had occurred in my life, I looked at that little piece of blue paper. "What's the big deal?" I thought. "Of course, reality is! Every idiot knows that!" It felt as though I had written "water is wet" and, for some reason, thought the insight was profound. Here, for the first time, I had encountered the limitations of language in trying to express mystical forms of consciousness. I meant to capture primal, eternal being, what the Christian theologian Paul Tillich called "The Ground of Being" or perhaps what Buddhists mean by "The Pure Land," something profoundly and intensely real that underlies the entire phenomenal, temporal world that most of us experience in everyday living. The words scratched on that scrap of blue paper were only an insipid souvenir from my first deep foray into transcendental forms of awareness.

So the words in this book, much as they are intended to communicate as comprehensively and accurately as my literary skills allow, sometimes demand patience and poetic license from you, the reader. I offer you my best as we explore the edges of an incredibly fascinating and important frontier, even though a voice within me would prefer simply to play music for you instead–perhaps Chopin Nocturnes with their many subtle nuances of emotional expression, or the profoundly powerful yet joyful and playful Fantasia and Fugue in G Minor by Johann Sebastian Bach.

ACKNOWLEDGMENTS

With gratitude, I acknowledge the primary mentors in my professional life: Huston Smith, Walter Houston Clark, Hanscarl Leuner, and Abraham Maslow, plus two whom I never had the honor to meet in person, Paul Tillich and Karl Jaspers.

Many colleagues have provided support over the years, sharing their own visions and dedication to fostering the responsible use of psychedelic substances. I especially acknowledge Charles Savage, Walter Pahnke, Stanislav Grof, Helen Bonny, Richard Yensen, and John Rhead from the days of research at the Spring Grove Hospital and the Maryland Psychiatric Research Center, and my current colleagues, Roland Griffiths, Mary Cosimano, Matthew Johnson, Margaret Kleindinst, Albert Garcia-Romeu, Frederick Barrett, Theresa Carbonaro, and Annie Umbricht from the States of Consciousness Research team at the Johns Hopkins School of Medicine. Robert Jesse, convener of the Council on Spiritual Practices, merits special recognition for his many skillfully orchestrated contributions to the rebirth of scientific investigations with these sacred substances.

On a personal level, I am thankful for the steady support of my primary companion in this phase of my life, the artist Edna Kurtz Emmet, and her two adult children, Nadav and Danielle. I honor my own two sons, Daniel and Brian, and their mother, Ilse, who for two decades prior to her death not only was my wife, but often also served as the psychiatric nurse who worked beside me in the implementation of various projects of psychedelic research. I am grateful for my parents, Ruth and Robert Richards, and my two brothers, Robert and John, who, even when they were rather bewildered by what I found of importance in my academic pursuits, continued to trust me as I followed my unique life trajectory.

The brilliant new generation of psychedelic researchers inspires me, including Stephen Ross, Anthony Bossis, Jeffrey Guss, Michael Bogenschutz, Paul Hutson, Karen Cooper, Randall Brown, Peter Hendricks, Michael and Annie Mithoefer, James Grigsby, Franz Vollenweider, Torsten Passie, Jordi Riba, José Carlos Bouso, Peter Gasser, Peter Oehen, Robin Carhart-Harris, David Nutt, David Erritzoe, and many others. Also, I express my gratitude and indebtedness to those who have provided private funding in support of ongoing research through the Heffter Research Institute and the Council on Spiritual Practices, and also the Fetzer Institute, and the Betsy Gordon Foundation, Beckley Foundation, and Riverstyx Foundation.

With profound appreciation, I recognize the hundreds of research volunteers and psychotherapy clients who have invited me into the depths of their lives and shared their unique struggles and transformative experiences. Each of them has influenced my life and thought.

There are many inspiring and innovative friends and companions in the steadily expanding psychedelic research community who contribute in their own ways. Luis Eduardo Luna, James Fadiman, Thomas Roberts, Charles Grob, Alicia Danforth, Rick Doblin, Neal Goldsmith, Iker Puente, Ben Sessa, David Nichols, George Greer, Dennis McKenna, Julie Holland, Amanda Feilding, Gabor Maté, Joshua Wickerham, and my son, Brian Richards, immediately come to mind. Authors who have combined scholarship and courageous creativity, such as Jeremy Narby, Michael Pollan, and Simon Powell, deserve explicit appreciation. Bimonthly lunches with my friend Allan Gold, complete with sushi or Nepalese cuisine, also have been enriching. My late friend Wayne Teasdale, who loved to meditate more than anyone I have ever met, merits special acknowledgment. And to Wendy Lochner, my editor from Columbia University Press, who intuited that I had a book within me that needed birthing and who has provided skilled guidance in its formation and composition, I offer profound appreciation. With her encouragement I have endeavored to write in a style that will be comprehensible to a wide readership, rather than to address the book in a traditional academic format to professional colleagues in either the mental health or religious communities.

Finally, since this book is about encountering the sacred and the discovery of eternal realms in consciousness, it also is appropriate to acknowledge that creative source that brought all of us into being, sustains our lives, and perhaps takes delight in the adventures of our ideas and our continuing evolution, here and now.

INTRODUCTION

This book is a humble offering of knowledge and perspectives that I have been privileged to gradually acquire, having had the unique opportunity to participate in the implementation of legal research projects with psychedelic drugs for over twenty-five years of my professional life. The incredibly rich variety of human volunteers I have accompanied and supported during the amazingly different states of consciousness that can be facilitated by these mind-manifesting substances have included men and women between the ages of twenty-four and eighty-one, varying in racial, educational, occupational, national, and religious backgrounds. Some have been suffering from anxiety, depression, and other manifestations of psychological distress. Others have been persons whose lives have been limited by addictions to alcohol or narcotic drugs. Still others have been persons with rapidly advancing cancer who are coming to terms with the lives they have lived and the imminence of death.

And volunteers have also included professional leaders in the fields of mental health and religion, as well as others from many different occupations who have asked to participate in research studies out of a yearning for personal, educational, or spiritual development. Almost all of these diverse volunteers had no prior personal experience with psychedelic substances and would not have been interested in participation were it not under legal, medical auspices. Thus they neither would have identified with any countercultural group nor would have been interested in what has come to be called recreational drug use. So it is that this book has emerged from the psychedelic experiences of very ordinary people who have been well engaged in the mainstream of life.

I write as a clinical psychologist with formal academic training that also included studies in theology, comparative religions, and the psychology of religion. I also write as a psychotherapist with a broadly based orientation that often could be labeled as existential or transpersonal. Like many readers, I have asked deep questions, have quested for meaning, and have sought to comprehend the processes of personal growth amid the inevitable struggles that most of us share in everyday existence. Since I have had the good fortune to personally receive psychedelic substances in legal contexts and find myself free to share some of the experiential knowledge thereby acquired, the source materials for this book have arisen not only from observations gleaned from research volunteers and the scientific analyses of data, but also from discoveries within the corridors of my own mind.

The cache of knowledge expressed in the pages ahead, both experiential and scientific, includes insights about human existence and the struggles and suffering most of us experience. It describes processes that foster healing and provide meaning, including some that may facilitate spiritual awakening. The discoveries made by the hundreds of persons whom I have encountered in the depths of their psychological and spiritual lives have profound relevance for beginning to more fully comprehend who we are, who we may become, and perhaps what the ultimate nature of reality may be. This collection of observations and experiences is of relevance not only for philosophers, psychologists, anthropologists, theologians, microbiologists, neuroscientists, and quantum physicists, but also for each of us who discovers himself or herself in the process that Buddhists call "one precious human life." As will be apparent as the content of this book unfolds, this growing edge of science also is a frontier of religious and spiritual knowledge.

A secondary intention is to provide information that may serve to more fully educate readers about what an increasing number of thoughtful and critical people believe to be the remarkable promise of psychedelic substances, when they are responsibly administered and ingested. This knowledge can dispel more of the distorted remnants of the sensationalistic press of the 1960s that continue to influence attitudes in the medical, religious, and political communities as well as in the population at large. These attitudes, often based on ignorance, distorted information, unrestrained passion to combat drug abuse, and legislative decisions that have disregarded the findings of sober science, have become manifested in public policies in national and international arenas that have forbidden or discouraged exploration of this frontier.

During the forty-five-year period of the so-called drug war, which some now call the war on some drugs or the plant war, the understanding of the man on the street appears to have become increasingly skewed. For many people the term "psychedelic," which simply means "mind-manifesting," has become all but indelibly associated with tie-dyed T-shirts, rose-colored glasses, rebellious behavior, and the risks associated with drug abuse. The insightful and inspiring writings about psychedelics by serious scholars such as Aldous Huxley, Alan Watts, and Huston Smith have almost been forgotten. Too often, young explorers of the mind, plagued by impulsiveness and misinformation (if not pills of questionable composition), have ended up in emergency rooms, courtrooms, and sometimes prisons. More mature users of psychedelics have tended to be more discrete, maintaining the privacy of their experiences out of fear of social censure and adverse impacts on their careers.

It is my hope that the range and depth of experiences presented in this book, along with the principles of maximizing the safety and potential benefit of psychedelic use, will prove helpful to readers who seek to more fully comprehend their own experiences in alternative states of consciousness, regardless of how they may have been facilitated, as well as those of friends and family members. Perhaps this information may also serve to catalyze our thinking about the origins of the powerful cultural taboo under which we have been living. Still further, this book may foster thoughtful deliberations about responsible and rational ways by which socially sanctioned access to these substances may be established to protect the freedom of those who have acquired adequate knowledge of potential risks and benefits and who desire to legally explore the "inner space" of their own minds with the respectful use of entheogens.

In lieu of footnotes, the reference style employed in this book provides sufficient information in the main text to enable the reader to locate supplemental information and sources in the bibliography. It provides a carefully chosen listing of relevant articles, books, and documentary films for further discernment and enjoyment by readers who find themselves motivated to explore particular topics in greater depth.

Now at age seventy-four, as I look back on my life, I realize that, like others near my age, I have lived through a remarkable period of social change. Not long ago, had someone told me that the Soviet Union would cease to exist, that the Berlin Wall would come down, that a president with brown skin would occupy the White House in Washington for two terms, or that women and gay and lesbian citizens would be approaching full equality, I would have tended to say, "Be real; live in the real world." Having participated in the original emergence, the repressive period of dormancy, and the reemergence of psychedelic research, including the many lessons learned during this dramatic saga that enhance the probability of safety and benefit, I find I have information to share that may help to pave the way for modifications in the current drug laws in the United States, in the United Kingdom, and in other countries. Beyond encouraging legislation that may culminate in new guidelines for research and medical, educational, and religious use, it is my hope that this book may serve to catalyze the many urgently needed projects of responsible research with these substances that have yet to be designed and implemented. As I stated in my first published article, coauthored with my friend Walter Pahnke in 1966, "a significant danger confronting our society may lie in losing out on the benefits that the responsible use of these drugs may offer."

NOTE TO THE READER

The information provided in this book is for educational, historical, and cultural interest only and should not be construed as advocacy for the current use of psychedelic substances under any circumstances outside settings where their use is legally sanctioned, such as for legal scientific research. Neither the author nor the publisher assumes any responsibility for physical, psychological, legal, or other consequences arising from the use of these substances.

SACRED KNOWLEDGE

PART I

Setting the Stage

The Death and Rebirth
of Psychedelic Research

Research with these unique substances thrived in many academic laboratories and psychotherapy treatment centers from the mid-1950s into the early 1970s. In the mid-1960s alone, over one thousand publications appeared that supported the promise of LSD in safely deepening and accelerating psychotherapy. Some forty thousand persons participated in these studies. Six international conferences were convened.

Then, in an irrational response to the turmoil of cultural pressures, including controversies about the war in Vietnam and shifting social mores, notably in the domains of race relations, the women's movement, and sexuality, perhaps also colored by the misguided attempts of the US Central Intelligence Agency to explore the military potential of LSD in interrogations or warfare, psychedelic research was rendered totally dormant by governmental action in the United States for twenty-two years (with the exception of one truncated study with DMT at the University of New Mexico between 1990 and 1995). Similar cessation of research occurred in the United Kingdom and in most other countries in accordance with UN treaties in 1971 and 1988. Unwittingly, in an impulsive desire to curb the use, misuse, and abuse of many different drugs, the promise of psychedelic substances in medicine–not to mention their potential roles in education and religion–was rendered dormant. It became all but impossible for qualified researchers to obtain the required approvals from federal agencies and local Institutional Review Boards to obtain, manufacture, or possess psychedelic substances and to conduct investigations with human volunteers.

In 1977, after administering psilocybin to a final volunteer in a study designed to decrease the psychological distress of cancer patients, I had the dubious distinction of being the last to leave the sinking ship at the Maryland Psychiatric Research Center, which, in turn, had become the only site in the United States where ongoing psychedelic research had been permitted to continue. The final deathblow, incidentally, came not from the federal government in Washington, but from university administrators who chose to focus state resources on less controversial areas of research. The findings of the many psychedelic research studies at this primary site were summarized by Richard Yensen and Donna Dryer, more or less lovingly placed in a time capsule for future investigators, and finally published in the 1994 Yearbook of the European College for the Study of Consciousness.

However, since the initiation of studies in Baltimore at the Johns Hopkins School of Medicine in 1999, spearheaded by Roland Griffiths and myself, and increasingly at other academic centers in North America and Western Europe, psychedelic research is now undergoing a promising surge of rebirth. Persons currently empowered to soberly weigh research evidence and to guide public policy, even those who themselves chose not to experiment with psychedelic drugs during their college years, have tended to think and act reasonably with openness and clarity. In the United States, the challenge to obtain the requisite Investigational New Drug Permit (IND) for a substance listed in Schedule I, along with approvals of research proposals from the Food and Drug Administration (FDA) and the Drug Enforcement Administration (DEA), requires high standards of scholarly competence and extreme patience, but it once again has become possible. As the first studies in this new wave of research have been published in professional journals, most writers and newscasters have reported the results in a factual manner without the sensationalistic flair that characterized much of the press coverage a few decades earlier.

The first of our studies at Johns Hopkins entailed a comparison of the alternate states of consciousness facilitated by the entheogen psilocybin and those evoked by a stimulant, methylphenidate (Ritalin), with thirty healthy adult residents of the Baltimore-Washington area who had no prior history of psychedelic drug use. Many of these people had known college friends or others who had experimented with psychedelic substances, but had personally chosen to wait until there might be a legal opportunity to receive them in known purity and dosage with competent guidance. When they heard about the Hopkins research project, they applied to participate. All experimental sessions were conducted individually with two research guides and one volunteer subject present in a comfortable space designed as a living room. There, each participant reclined on a couch, usually wearing a sleep-shade to prevent environmental distractions and headphones that provided supportive music during most of the six-hour period of drug action.

In accordance with the current standards of research in psychopharmacology, the study was designed and implemented with double-blind methods, meaning that no one other than the pharmacist who filled the opaque, blue capsules, identical in appearance, knew whether the contents prescribed for a particular volunteer on a particular day happened to be psilocybin or Ritalin. Thus, everything was held constant except for the prescribed substance. The screening interviews, the preparation and expectations, the behavior of the research personnel, the choice of music played during the periods of drug action, and the questionnaires and assessment tools employed all were standardized. After the drug effects abated, each volunteer completed questionnaires that surveyed the degree to which a broad range of alternative states of awareness and concomitant cognitive, emotional, and somatic responses had occurred.

When the results were analyzed, one-third of those who received psilocybin rated their inner experiences as the most spiritually significant of their lives, whereas no such claims of similar confidence and intensity were made by those who received Ritalin. More than two-thirds of the participants who received psilocybin rated their experiences as among the five most important events of their lives, akin to the birth of a child or the death of a parent. In follow-up interviews and assessments by close friends and family members fourteen months after the psilocybin experiences, reports of enduring positive life changes were supported. Subsequent studies have yielded similar findings. Detailed research information and published results on these and other projects can be found in the bibliography of this book and also on the world wide web, conveniently on the websites of the Council on Spiritual Practices (csp.org/psilocybin) and Erowid (erowid.org).

Now approximately 250 volunteers have received psilocybin at Hopkins alone. There is no question in my mind that, when used in accordance with medical guidelines, with skilled preparation and guidance in responsibly monitored, legal environments, psilocybin and similar substances are indeed molecules that can facilitate beneficial and often sacred experiences. The available evidence strongly indicates that they can be administered safely by well-informed researchers or by trained mental health and religious professionals to many people who desire to employ these sacramental tools in their pursuit of personal and spiritual growth. It also remains true that, when used irresponsibly with insufficient knowledge, these substances can facilitate experiences that may have negative consequences for some persons.

Before the Controlled Substances Act was passed by the US Congress during the Nixon Administration in 1970, which placed most psychedelic substances in the highly restricted Category I (that is, drugs with no accepted medical use in the United States, that are considered to have high abuse potential, and about which there is a lack of agreement regarding safety under medical supervision), many well-respected scholars and religious leaders in the United States and around the world legally received them and freely wrote about the significance of their experiences. Aldous Huxley, Alan Watts, Huston Smith, Gerald Heard, Bill Wilson, Rabbi Zalman Schachter-Shalomi, and Brother David Steindl-Rast immediately come to mind.

One may also note the Nobel Prize–winning geneticists Francis Crick and Kary Mullis, along with Steve Jobs, the cofounder of Apple Computers, all of whom acknowledged the contribution of psychedelics to their creative processes. Similarly, the psychiatrists and psychologists who pursued research or clinical treatment with these substances in those days almost always arranged training experiences for themselves and their coworkers, which they openly acknowledged in periodic reports to the FDA, reasoning that it would have been difficult to comprehend the experiences of their patients and research subjects without personal, experiential knowledge. Such educational use was legal at that time because the drugs, then as now, were understood to be essentially nontoxic and nonaddictive. Meanwhile, in several indigenous cultures in Central and South America, in East Africa, and in the United States and Canada, men and women sacramentally incorporated the psychedelic substances contained in various cacti, mushrooms, shrubs, and vines as an intrinsic part of their spiritual disciplines, as many have done since the dawn of man, continuing today. Native Americans are thought to have used mescaline for spiritual purposes for as long as fifty-five hundred years. Cave paintings of human-like figures with mushrooms have been found on the Tassili Plateau in Northern Algeria, dated to 5000 BCE.

In spite of the legal sanctions imposed since 1970, some so severe as to merit the adjective "draconian," many contemporary people throughout the world who are not official members of indigenous religious groups or participants in research projects approved by the FDA or similar governmental authorities in other countries still have chosen to ingest psychedelic substances. Their reasons have varied, ranging from youthful or professional curiosity, to the search for relief from symptoms of emotional distress, to the hope of facilitating creativity, to the thirst for religious and spiritual knowledge. A recent survey by two Norwegian researchers, Teri Krebs and Pål-Orjan Johansen, based on 2010 data, estimated thirty-two million current residents in the United States alone who have used psilocybin, LSD, or mescaline. The Drug Policy Alliance in 2014 estimated the number of citizens who have used psychedelics in the United States at thirty-four million.

At the time of writing, ongoing research with human volunteers and psychedelic substances is taking place, not only at the Johns Hopkins School of Medicine, but also at an increasing number of other sites, including New York University, the University of California in Los Angeles, the University of New Mexico, Harvard University, the University of Wisconsin, and the University of Alabama, as well as at the Imperial College in London and in Canada, Germany, Switzerland, Israel, Spain, Mexico, and New Zealand. For those who deeply believe in the promise of these sacred substances, in medicine, in education, or in religion, it is a hopeful time.

2

Orientation, Definitions, and the Limits of Language

PREPARATION FOR EXPLORING CONSCIOUSNESS

Much as I have personally come to value the major psychedelic substances, to view them as intrinsically sacred, and to believe in their promise to constructively contribute to the quality of life on our planet when people utilize them in intelligent ways, I affirm at the outset that they are but one of many tools that may be employed in the process of human psychological and spiritual development. These substances are regarded especially highly by many different people, not simply because busy Westerners may tend to be impatient in their spiritual quests, but also because entheogens, wisely ingested, are noted for their power and effectiveness, thereby potentially supplementing other psychological and spiritual disciplines. For those who may choose to include these substances in their personal, religious, or professional lives, it is hoped in contexts that are legal and well structured in the not too distant future, the acquisition of knowledge about potential risks and careful preparation are as critically important as it would be for someone deciding to take the risks involved in many other ventures and adventures.

For example, consider downhill skiing: I recall a beautiful, crisp winter day in my early twenties when I decided to finally go skiing.

Without any instruction, I rented a pair of skis at a scenic lodge in the Harz Mountains in Germany, slid my feet into their binders, and started down a modest slope, trying to keep my feet parallel. An attractive girl coming up the slope smiled at me and softly said "schön" (beautiful). My speed and my pride at not having fallen yet gradually increased. Suddenly, with dismay I saw that I was headed straight toward a large group of people at the bottom of the hill and realized that I had no knowledge of how to steer, slow down, or stop. After a few futile seconds of trying to keep calm and think logically, I desperately leapt into the air and tumbled into a heap in the snow, fortunately still being young and flexible enough not to break any bones.

Embarrassed, I then tried to climb back to the top of the slope, pushing forward and immediately sliding backward, barely advancing as sweet little children smiled and tromped on past me. Amid the impulsiveness, arrogance, and ignorance that endanger many of us when we are young, I had put both myself and others at risk. I learned some humility that day, and subsequently sought out some basic instruction on the art of skiing. I credit myself with having had sufficient good judgment not to have begun on a double black-diamond slope, but the truth is that I wasn't ready on that day for any slope at all. The day did come, however, when, as the sun was rising, I could ride a cable car to the top of a mountain, glide through peaceful, pine forests in solitary meditation, gradually meet others as trails converged, and finally arrive safe and invigorated at a lodge deep in the valley below.

As will become progressively clear in the chapters ahead, the use of psychedelic substances is also an art that requires some skills. There are principles of navigation in the inner world that can be taught and learned. Much more is involved in facilitating life-enhancing experiences with these incredible molecules than simply swallowing a capsule, pill, or piece of blotter paper, drinking some tea, or chewing on some plant material and then awaiting "drug effects." In passing, however, permit me to register the thoughts that we do not make skiing illegal because some people injure themselves or others, and that there are many who really love to ski, do it skillfully and responsibly, and find it life-enhancing. Still skiing is not for everyone, and there are those who for medical or psychological reasons, or for pure lack of interest and motivation, may be well advised to explore other life activities instead.

MYSTICAL CONSCIOUSNESS

The core of this book is about the nature and relevance of mystical consciousness and the visionary experiences that sometimes precede, follow, or accompany this unspeakably vast, dynamic, magnificent, and profoundly meaningful state of awareness. (Please forgive the many adjectives, but, as some readers already understand, they honestly underemphasize the true reality of this form of consciousness.) Although the meaning of terms like "mystical" and "visionary" will be carefully defined and discussed in detail, let it be clear from the outset that "mystical" has nothing to do with states of mind that are misty or vague. Nor does the term refer to magic or usual occult or paranormal phenomena.

Rather this term denotes a form of consciousness that vividly remains in the memory banks of those who witness it (or claim to die into it and be reborn afterward) that goes by many names, such as "Ultimate Reality," "Cosmic Consciousness," "The Eternal Core of Being," or the "Source of the Perennial Philosophy." All of the great world religions have words that point toward this highly desired and valued state of spiritual awareness, such as *samadhi* in Hinduism, *nirvana* in Buddhism, *sekhel mufla* in Judaism, *the beatific vision* in Christianity, *baqá wa faná* in Islam, and *wu wei* in Taoism. Although there may well be room for infinite variations in the nature and descriptions of individual reports of these experiences, which have delighted scholars of mystical literature and researchers of meditative states of consciousness in years past and will continue to occupy them long into the future, the research with psychedelic substances surveyed in this book strongly supports the reality of a common core of characteristics and the validity of what Robert K. C. Forman has called the "Pure Consciousness Event," or PCE. This "common core" reliably includes descriptions of (1) Unity, (2) Transcendence of Time and Space, (3) Intuitive Knowledge, (4) Sacredness, (5) Deeply-Felt Positive Mood, and (6) Ineffability, all experiential categories that subsequently will be explored in depth.

Some recent scholars of religious experience, represented by Steven T. Katz from Boston University, have argued against the reality of a universal state of consciousness at the "core" or "ground" of being that has been discovered and rediscovered perennially by people from different cultures throughout history. Calling themselves "constructivists," they have posited that the experiences people call revelatory or religious are significantly influenced or predetermined by their expectations, language, styles of thinking, and systems of belief. Religious experiences have thus been viewed as crafted or constructed by the implicit suggestions inherent in one's community and culture. In contrast, they have tended to depict the "perennialist view," expressed by such scholars as Aldous Huxley in *The Perennial Philosophy*, Walter Stace in *Mysticism and Philosophy*, and Edward Kelly in *Irreducible Mind* and critically discussed by the psychologist of religion Ralph Hood as an archaic idea from the distant twentieth century. The evidence presented in this book represents a strong swing of the theoretical pendulum back toward the so-called perennialist perspective. This does not deny that some experiences and their interpretation are colored by expectations and suggestions. However, as simply expressed in the words of the theologian Paul Tillich, it appears that there may actually be a "really real God." Some may prefer to use nouns other than the three English letters of "g-o-d" to refer to this reality, from either religious or scientific vocabularies, but there is good reason to affirm that there is indeed an eternal dimension of awareness deep in the core of the human mind where creativity, love, and beauty reign supreme. In Tillich's words from *Biblical Religion and the Search for Ultimate Reality*:

> If we enter the levels of personal existence which have been rediscovered by depth psychology, we encounter the past, the ancestors, the collective unconscious, the living substance in which all living beings participate. In our search for the "really real" we are driven from one level to another to a point where we cannot speak of level any more, where we must ask for that which is the ground of all levels, giving them their structure and their power of being.

Beyond the active "asking" of our inquisitive intellects, yearning to comprehend the nature of reality and our place within it, is the passive receiving and discovery of the realms of truth we call spiritual and eternal within the states of consciousness we call revelatory and mystical.

A VARIETY OF APPROACHES

The major psychedelic substances employed in the research on which this book is based include psilocybin, LSD (d-lysergic acid diethylamide), DPT (dipropyltryptamine), MDA (methylenedioxyamphetamine), and DMT (dimethyltryptamine). However, this is a book not about "drug experiences" per se, but rather about the profoundly meaningful states of consciousness that they may occasion when employed with knowledge and skill. It is my conclusion that these incredibly beautiful, awe-inspiring, and, for some, terrifying experiences are best understood not as being "within the drugs," but rather as being within our own minds.

These unique and fascinating states of consciousness can also be facilitated by many nondrug approaches, though sometimes yielding experiential discoveries that for many appear to be less vivid in intensity or completeness. This includes a plethora of meditative techniques from different religious traditions, many of which include focused attention coupled with changes in breathing patterns that alter the balance of oxygen and carbon dioxide in the blood. Some people may prefer sensory isolation, sitting in perfectly quiet spaces or being suspended in dark tanks of saltwater at body temperature. Others may opt for sensory flooding or overload while immersing themselves in the music of rock bands or symphony orchestras. Mystical and visionary experiences are sometimes encountered during natural childbirth, religious rituals, communion with nature, or exceptional sexual orgasms, or while deeply engaged in feats of personal athletic or artistic performance. Often they appear to occur unintentionally, whether brought about by stress, concentration, sleep deprivation, fasting, diet, or concomitant changes in our own brain chemistry, or by the action of what many believe to be divine grace.

What makes the responsible use of psychedelic substances so important, however, is that it provides *reliability* and *potency*. For the first time in the history of science, these two factors allow these revelatory states of consciousness and any changes in physical or mental health, or in attitudes or behavior, that may follow them to be studied carefully and systematically within the context of academic research. No longer is the study of mysticism limited to the scholarly scrutiny of historical documents, such as the beautifully expressive writings of St. Teresa of Avila, Meister Eckhart, Rumi, or Shankara. Nor is it limited to the noble attempts to express the subtle shifts of awareness encountered in meditative disciplines within the structural limitations of human language. Profoundly sacred experiences are now occurring in the laboratories of medical professionals and social scientists.

THE MYSTERY THAT WE ARE

Expanded into a larger perspective, the issue of the relationship of these particular molecular compounds to inner experiential content fades into the enigmatic question of the relationship of the human nervous system to consciousness, and perhaps still further into the mystery of matter itself, those atomic and subatomic energies that form the cells of our bodies and brains and dance within and between them. Pierre Teilhard de Chardin (1881–1955), the Jesuit paleontologist who suggested that we are actually all spiritual beings who are currently having physical or human experiences, called matter "the divine milieu." He described a powerful mystical experience of his own in a poetic essay titled "The Spiritual Power of Matter," published in *Hymn of the Universe*, including these lines: "Son of man, bathe yourself in the ocean of matter; plunge into it where it is deepest and most violent; struggle in its currents and drink of its waters. For it cradled you long ago in your preconscious existence; and it is that ocean that will raise you up to God." For those who like to quote scriptures, the words of St. Paul in his first letter to the young church in Corinth merit reflection: "For the temple of God is holy; and that is what you are" (1 Cor. 3:17).

A psychologist colleague of mine, Roland Fischer, in order to remind himself of how little we really know, always kept on the left rear corner of his desk a framed photograph of a monkey staring wide-eyed at his own image in a mirror and scratching his head. Profound questions arise for all of us who wonder what we might really be and who eventually must come to terms with death. Those who have experienced mystical consciousness almost universally report that they find the reductionist assumptions of many scientists and nonscientists, who tend to simply assume that consciousness is caused by brain activity alone, to be less than compelling. In spite of the fascinating advances being made in neuroscience, linking mental states with chemical changes, electrical activity, or alterations of blood flow and oxygen content in certain areas of the human brain, correlation is not necessarily causation.

Among alternative theoretical approaches is the philosophy of Henri Bergson, a French philosopher popular in the early twentieth century, recently reintroduced by G. William Barnard, who viewed the brain as a reducing valve, akin to a television set that may modify or selectively focus content that does not originate within itself. Similarly, one may reflect on the wise caution of Tenzin Gyatso, His Holiness, the 14th Dalai Lama, who, in his book *The Universe in a Single Atom*, wrote that "the view that all mental processes are necessarily physical processes is a metaphysical assumption, not a scientific fact," and observed that current neuroscience does not have "any real explanation of consciousness itself." Karl Jaspers, a German psychiatrist and philosopher who, with his Jewish wife Gertrud, suffered through World War II, repetitively reminded the readers of his many books that we are fundamentally more than we know or perhaps ever can know of ourselves. When we attempt to organize vivid descriptions or actual memories of mystical and visionary experiences within the filing systems of our rational minds, we find that our current linguistic skills and cognitive categories are still very primitive.

We have languages from different academic disciplines, each with their growing edges, that may strive to approach and articulate the mystery of consciousness. Biochemistry may attempt to describe molecular and electrical transmissions at somewhere around one hundred trillion synapses within our nervous systems. Neuroscience strives to point to pathways and patterns of activity involving about one billion neurons, changes in blood flow within our brains, and alterations of oxygen consumption by our cells. Physics may point to the activity of quanta of energy and even identify photons emitted by our DNA. All knowledge of this nature illumines the amazing complexity of our lives. One may find beauty as well as new insights and discoveries in the microscopic and submicroscopic structures and processes we are beginning to uncover.

In beginning to decipher this mystery, for example, we may value knowing that psilocybin rapidly metabolizes into psilocin, which, like the neurotransmitter serotonin, binds with 5-H2A receptors in our brains, and that blood flow and oxygen content in our medial prefrontal and posterior cingulate cortices and in our thalami, areas referred to as our "default mode networks," appear to decrease when psilocin is facilitating the occurrence of alternate states of consciousness. Jeremy Narby has boldly speculated that some of the incredibly intricate geometric patterns discovered during the action of entheogens might actually be microscopic cellular structures somehow being perceived through an as yet unidentified, inner-directed visionary capacity that we all may possess.

Yet it does not suffice to describe a revelatory insight as a mere electrical impulse or an emotion as the squirt of a hormone. Love, nobility, the creative yearnings to strive toward and express excellence, and what we humans call "greatness" are manifestations of that part of the mystery of our beings that we call "spiritual." The same is true of dedication and courage to care about our human foibles and the commitments we make to work toward the resolution of personal, societal, and international impasses. The mystics, past and present, are not only those who have glimpsed an ultimate eternal harmony and somehow managed to remember it; many of them are also known to have returned to the simple disciplines of everyday existence, to "chop wood and carry water," that is, to have become incarnate in the world and grounded within time. Perhaps the most highly evolved minds among us come close to genuinely living in both worlds, the eternal and the temporal. In the language of Christian theology, this could be seen to mirror, however faintly, the archetype of the Christ who is fully divine and fully human, capable of experiencing both the agony of crucifixion and the joy of resurrection. In the language of Buddhist theology, the bodhisattva humbly walks the streets of the marketplace dedicated to compassionate involvement in serving others.

NONMYSTICAL FORMS OF PSYCHEDELIC EXPERIENCE

It is important to realize that a substantial number of people have ingested psychedelic drugs on many occasions without experiencing the profound states of consciousness explored in this book. These substances, especially when they are ingested in low dosage without an understanding of powerful factors such as trust, honesty, courage, and openness in environments not conducive to safe introspection, can provide changes in sensory perception and mild forms of mental imagery that may be experienced as either delightful or frightening.

They can also trigger personal psychological experiences, such as regression to childhood traumas or confrontation with unresolved grief, fear, anger, or guilt. Such experiences, as will be discussed later, may well have potentially significant value in accelerating psychotherapy and personal growth, whether or not they are viewed as having religious import. Further, especially if one is unprepared and seeks to control or escape from emerging inner experiences, the flow of unique mental adventures facilitated by psychedelic substances can culminate in episodes of panic, paranoia, confusion, and somatic distress and perhaps a trip to an emergency room for psychiatric care. None of these "psychedelic experiences" are visionary or mystical as these terms are defined in the pages ahead.

There is no generic state of consciousness following the ingestion of these compounds that could be labeled "*the* psychedelic experience," just as we know there is no singular meditation experience, religious experience, or psychotherapeutic experience. Yet, as will become progressively clear, this does not imply that the effects of these substances should be viewed as unpredictable or capricious. Given knowledge of the many different factors that influence each individual psychedelic experience, the mental phenomena that occur for a particular person on a particular day often reflect remarkable coherence and meaning.

PERSONAL PRIVACY AND MYSTICAL EXPERIENCES

The psychologist Abraham Maslow (1908–1970), a natural Jewish mystic who never took psychedelic drugs and one of my esteemed mentors, called profound mystical states "peak experiences." He found that they spontaneously occurred in the lives of highly creative persons that he considered "self-actualizing," such as Albert Einstein and Eleanor Roosevelt. Many readers treasure memories of such experiences, regardless of how they may have been facilitated. They tend to provide a deep sense of inner security and often constitute a source of strength during periods of suffering or struggle in life and as one approaches death. As skillfully portrayed by Hermann Hesse in his short novel *Journey to the East*, it is often hard to recognize the enlightened minds around us. Sometimes, instead of being highly credentialed academic or religious leaders, they may well turn out to be your garbage man, a cleaning lady, or the checkout clerk at the supermarket.

Those who have known these profoundly meaningful states of consciousness have often shared them with no one, or only with those most intimately trusted, for fear of being misunderstood, called crazy or weird, or viewed as mentally ill. It is my hope that the experiences and perspectives presented in this book will enable such readers to realize that they are not alone and to trust their own revelatory glimpses of deeper levels of reality with more confidence and peace, even when they are unsure which words they might choose, were they to attempt to describe them. As Maslow believed, these experiences may be viewed as forays into "the higher reaches of human nature" rather than as symptoms of psychopathology.

For those who have not yet deeply probed into the depths or heights of their minds, perhaps this book may foster appreciation and tolerance for those friends and family members who have experienced such incredible nonordinary states of consciousness. For mental health practitioners who have been wary of reports of religious experiences or who have tended to dismiss most of religious belief and behavior as naïve, immature, or pathological, perhaps this book may encourage appreciation for and openness to a more profound understanding of the spiritual dimension of human consciousness than they may have gleaned during their childhoods or formal academic training. For those who may tend to view the world through religious structures of thought that emphasize exclusiveness and the literal interpretation of scriptures, the content of this book may invite new insights into the many different ways in which the sacred becomes manifested in human awareness.

When peak experiences occur, they usually tend to be humbly received. Often they are interpreted as glimpses into domains of human consciousness beyond one's individual life, and thus, even as the memories may be treasured, they tend not to be viewed as personal possessions. What was experienced typically feels universal and "belongs to all." This is one more reason that those who have known these experiences tend to keep them private and often view them as precious.

REGARDING THE CHOICE OF WORDS

I tend to use the word "drug" judiciously as for many it seems to trigger associations with "being drugged," with its connotations of escapism from responsible engagement with the world and not "being in your right mind." Many religiously oriented people have looked skeptically at psychedelics, concerned that they might foster hedonistic indulgence rather than truly spiritual revelations. Similarly, those dedicated to addressing drug abuse in our culture, a social concern of critical importance, have sometimes tended to lump all drugs together in their anti-drug rhetoric, not even distinguishing between narcotics, sedatives, stimulants, and psychedelics. In the words of a narcotic addict treated with LSD-assisted psychotherapy: "As far as the comparison of heroin and LSD, there is none. LSD helps you to find yourself; heroin helps you to hide from all kinds of responsibilities and from life itself. LSD has more reality, because when you find yourself in it, you can live life better."

Most of us in Western cultures have a collection of drugs in our medicine cabinets and tend to expect receipt of a prescription or two when we visit our physicians, often for medications that have been promised to help us cope with anxiety or depression if taken regularly. In addition, whether responsibly or irresponsibly, many of us freely consume drugs such as caffeine, alcohol, nicotine, or marijuana. "Just say no," well intentioned as it once was when Nancy Reagan's words were incorporated into an advertising campaign supported by the National Institutes of Health, has been firmly countered in recent years by "just say know." It is past time for an educated populace to understand each substance and to come to know the distinction between responsible use and the misuse or abuse of each of them. It is my judgment that the average person is bright enough to master such knowledge, especially now with access to reliable information easily found on our cell phones via the Internet. There was a time, only a century ago, when many strongly believed that the human nervous system could not safely control automobiles at speeds faster than horses could gallop; now we zoom along multilaned expressways at high speeds, a few feet from one another, with reasonable grace and ease. We learn and we evolve.

But if I don't use the term "psychedelic drugs," what then are the alternatives? Some of my colleagues have opted for "psychedelic medicines," but medicines tend to be understood as treatments for sicknesses rather than catalysts of personal and spiritual growth. For this term to meaningfully resonate, one must understand our estrangement from the sacredness of nature, of ourselves and other people, and view our baseline human condition at this point in history as a "sickness" that may require a "medicine" for cure. This term and the perspective it reflects, however, are well established in some indigenous cultures where psychedelic substances are accepted as religious sacraments.

One could consider "psychedelic supplements," like natural herbs intended to promote good health, but this framework still implies a need for repetitive use. We now understand that the benefits of a well-planned psychedelic experience come not from the substance itself, but rather from the integration of the enduring memories of the particular states of consciousness that were experienced during the period of drug action. That is why those who encounter profoundly meaningful states of mind typically express little interest in repetitive ingestions in the near future.

Other alternatives in the research history of these substances include such proposed terms as "phantastica" (by Louis Lewin, the Prussian pharmacologist who published an analysis of the Peyote cactus in 1886), "psychotomimetics" (mimickers of psychoses), "mysticomimetics" (mimickers of mystical states), "psychodysleptics" (disturbers of mental activity), "psycholytics" (mind-releasers), Aldous Huxley's term "phanerothymes" (spirit manifestors), and recently Michael Winkelman's suggestion of "psychointegrators." The term "hallucinogens" still appears in most recent medical publications, but it is a misnomer since true hallucinations with these substances are exceedingly rare. Even when, during the action of a psychedelic substance, one may "see" the inner visionary world projected upon or incorporated within environmental perceptions, one usually maintains critical awareness and knows that those nearby cannot share in the same experiences.

The term "entheogen," coined in 1979 by Carl Ruck, a professor in Boston University's Classical Studies Department, has been growing in acceptance, meaning "generating God within." This focus is congruent with the primary theme of this book, though as noted there are many forms of experience triggered by psychedelic substances that are not "entheogenic," that is, they are not characterized by visionary or mystical content that most of us would view as having relevance for religion or spirituality. Also, the idea of "generating God" does not fit, since mystical consciousness is almost always experienced as a gift received, not as the result of human effort. "Discovering God within" would be more on target.

Considering all these options, I have opted to use the terms "entheogens" and "psychedelic substances" interchangeably. With these words, above all, I refer to psilocybin, the active ingredient in the mushrooms called sacred or magic that have been used by indigenous people in Mesoamerica in their religious and healing rites for perhaps three thousand years, if not longer, continuing today. Psilocybin has been the prime entheogen in our research at the Johns Hopkins School of Medicine during the past fifteen years. To control for purity and exact dosage, the psilocybin we have used has been synthesized in a pharmaceutical laboratory at Purdue University. Our pharmacists weigh it carefully and place it in blue capsules for volunteers in our various research projects. (I've often fantasized that, out of humor alone, a pharmacist someday might place a dose in a red capsule, but science is serious business and it has never happened!) The synthesized compound is similar, however, to natural "shrooms," any of over 180 different species of psilocybin-containing mushrooms that grow throughout the world and often appear in such diverse locations as the Olympic and Amazonian rain forests; throughout much of temperate Europe; in Australia, Tasmania, and New Zealand; in China, India, and Russia; on Mexican mountainsides; on the tundra of Siberia; in mason jars on college campuses and, I've been told, very mysteriously on courthouse lawns.

These terms, "entheogens" and "psychedelic substances," also may refer to mescaline, the active ingredient in the Peyote cactus used sacramentally by members of the Native American Church; to dimethyltryptamine (DMT), a substance active in the incredible brew called ayahuasca, sometimes administered weekly to the members of at least three religions in Brazil and neighboring countries; and to d-lysergic acid diethylamide (LSD), the molecule that the Swiss chemist Albert

Hofmann synthesized in 1938 and accidentally ingested in 1943 that still evokes such irrational responses, pro and con, that many researchers today hesitate even to mention it. One advantage of conducting research with psilocybin instead of LSD, besides its long natural history, its established safety profile, and its shorter duration of action, is frankly that the word is hard to spell and tends not to attract the press or evoke the emotionally labile reactions that commonly have been triggered by hearing the three letters "L-S-D." There are similar substances, such as dipropyltryptamine (DPT), diethyltryptamine (DET), methylenedioxyamphetamine (MDA), and many others discussed by the innovative chemist Alexander, or Sasha, Shulgin, recently deceased at age eighty-eight, in his books *PiHKAL* (which stands for "phenylethylamines I have known and loved") and *TiHKAL* (which stands for "tryptamines I have known and loved").

Another term I have avoided in this book is the familiar reference to altered states of consciousness. "Altered" seems to imply change from some idealized norm that may be considered a healthy baseline, and it also makes me think of how we take our cats and dogs to veterinarians to "get altered." It has the same prejudicial connotations as terms like "mind-bending," "distorting," or "artificial." When persons in my psychotherapy practice have expressed a yearning to be normal, I sometimes have responded, "Why would you want to do that?" The norm is the average in a society, and unfortunately normal behavior for many tends to be compulsively acquiring worldly goods, mindlessly watching television, and drinking beer—not necessarily an ideal to which we all should aspire.

Some of the states of consciousness considered in this book deviate from the norm, but that does not necessarily imply psychopathology. Whether or not Moses, Isaiah, Ezekiel, St. Paul, Muhammad, or Siddhartha Gautama should be viewed as being abnormal, or as having suffered from some variety of mental illness, when they experienced their visions may well constitute a subject for fascinating discussions in psychiatric, psychological, or theological classrooms. Two terms that I find more appropriate are "alternate" and "nonordinary," neither of which sounds especially judgmental.

A final term that merits clarification is the word "sacred." I use it without any necessarily implied connection to institutional forms of religion. Some readers may be more comfortable with the words "awe," "awesome," or "awe-inspiring." I refer to that intuitive sense of respectful, hushed sensitivity, often expressed in silence, that most people seem to experience when they enter a high nave of a Gothic cathedral or a spacious mosque with a beautiful interior dome. Perhaps the environmental perceptions somehow resonate intuitively within our nervous systems, evoking a feeling of reverence quite independent of whatever affiliations we may have with organized religious institutions. Some may encounter similar intuitive feelings when looking at the Milky Way on a clear night, when watching a spectacular sunrise or sunset, when holding the hand of a beloved person at the moment of death, or when first embracing a newborn child.

While on the subject of nomenclature, note also that I use the words "consciousness" and "mind" as synonyms, referring simply to our inner fields of awareness, including the totality of our perceptions, thoughts, mental images, emotions, intentions, and memories. The terms refer to what we observe, experience, and recall, whether with open or closed eyes, on a vast continuum between unconsciousness or dreamless sleep and that state of being fully awake that some seers would call Enlightenment. It could be described simply as "what we notice going on within us." Scholars of esoteric phenomena and some practitioners of alternative or complementary forms of medicine may make fine distinctions between words like "mind," "soul," "spirit," "psyche," "consciousness," "astral body," "etheric body," "subtle body," "chi body," and so forth, striving to carefully define what they intend to communicate with each term. Without devaluing such concepts, regardless of their potential utility or validity, no such distinctions are made or implied in the book at hand. I opt for simplicity, sort of a "meat and potatoes" approach to discussing the mysteries of our being.

FOCUS AND LIMITATIONS

Although pure MDMA (methylenedioxymethampetamine, sometimes contained in drugs called XTC, Molly, Mandy, or Ecstasy) may well become established as a valued substance in medicine, especially for use in couples counseling and the treatment of posttraumatic stress disorder, and though there are reports that it may occasionally facilitate mystical forms of experience for some people, it is considered more an "empathogen" or "entactogen" than an "entheogen," and thus is not included in the major psychedelic drugs on which this book is based. For readers interested in the ongoing research that may well eventually establish MDMA as a prescription medicine for traumatized veterans and others, current information can be found on the website of the Multidisciplinary Association for Psychedelic Studies (maps.org). Other reliable information can be found in books by Julie Holland and Sean Leneghan. For people who tend to be very anxious or who have difficulty trusting others or their own minds, it has been suggested that an initial experience with MDMA might constitute helpful preparation for a session with one of the major psychedelic substances.

Similarly, I have essentially no personal knowledge about Ibogaine, the substance used religiously by the Bwiti people in Central East Africa that may prove to be uniquely effective in the treatment of narcotic addiction. This also applies to the anesthetic Ketamine, Salvia divinorum, 2 C-B, and many similar recently synthesized substances about which I do not feel qualified to address either their potential benefits or the physiological or psychological risks that may be incurred in their use.

From observing the range of experiences reported by research volunteers with the major entheogens mentioned, I have concluded that it is reasonable to view these psychedelic substances as different skeleton or universal keys that can unlock the door within each of our minds to other forms of consciousness, essentially providing an opportunity for exploration and discovery rather than a particular discrete form of experience. There is a lot of lore, both in professional circles and on the streets, about how specific substances may evoke specific experiences, whether visions of particular deities, of elves or dragons, of glimpses of life in Medieval Europe, of alien life forms, or of how the world may have appeared at the age of two. People who have taken a particular dose of a particular substance and encountered a particular state of consciousness have often tended to conclude that whatever they happen to have experienced is "what that substance does."

In truth, if any substance in defined purity and dosage indeed has a higher probability than others of evoking specific strata of experiencing, that will only be demonstrated in future well-designed, double-blind projects of research in which neither the volunteer nor the accompanying guide knows the specific substance or dosage administered. In my experience, the range of alternative states of consciousness facilitated by LSD, DPT, psilocybin, and DMT is very similar, if not identical. The substances primarily appear to differ from one another in terms of speed of onset, arc and length of action, and abruptness of returning one to the everyday world.

I anticipate that some of the perspectives expressed in this book will evoke questions and discussion that, in turn, I hope will become manifested in scholarly debate and well-designed projects of empirical research in the future. I freely acknowledge that the content in the pages ahead is influenced by my own particular collection of life experiences, with and without psychedelic substances, within the corridors of my own mind and in interaction with other people. However, I know that very similar, if not identical, perspectives have also been reported by many of the research volunteers and professional colleagues with whom I have interacted over the years. Together, we have arrived on the edge of an awesomely vast frontier. It is my hope that our knowledge, supplemented by those who will continue this quest to comprehend uncharted terrains of the human mind after our deaths, will continue to expand in ever-greater scope and clarity.

INEFFABILITY AND LANGUAGE

Books, such as the one that you hold in your hand in either paper or digital form, are collections of words—written symbols or squiggles that can be expressed in spoken sounds. This one happens to be originally written in the form of English that is current in the early twenty-first century. We attempt to communicate accurately with one another by using words as skillfully as possible to share information or experiences. Especially when it comes to the attempt to share profoundly personal and meaningful human experiences, words sometimes seem woefully inadequate, and we may wonder if a gesture, a poem, a musical phrase, or a few abstract lines on a blank canvas might prove more effective.

When it comes to communicating mystical forms of consciousness, perhaps the most personal and meaningful experiences in the human repertoire, words seem especially limiting. The seer who wrote the Tao Tê Ching, an ancient Chinese Taoist Scripture, captured this frustration well in the verse, "He who knows does not speak; he who speaks does not know." Similarly, the nineteenth-century Russian poet Fyodor Tyutchev wrote simply that, when trying to speak about mystical experiences, "a word that's spoken is a lie." Research volunteers who find mystical consciousness in their memory banks when they emerge from the alternate states of awareness occasioned by psychedelic substances usually comply with their prior agreements to write a descriptive report of all they can recall, but invariably they also protest that the required task is almost hopeless and that the essence of their experiences remains inexpressible.

One factor in ineffability appears simply to be a lack of vocabulary. People claim to have experienced content in visionary worlds for which we have no words. Sometimes they have felt themselves immersed in another culture, even another time period in the distant past or perhaps even in the future. It's been likened to how a caveman might respond were he suddenly transported into Manhattan today, surrounded by skyscrapers, subways, jetliners, and people texting on cell phones. When, upon return to his cave, were his wife to ask, "Gorg, what did you experience?," all the poor man could do is grunt, and perhaps say that it was big, loud, and impressive. He might even have used a term like "awesome." Yet he could well have an intuitive impression that what he experienced had a logical structure within which there were processes that might well be articulated by some future generation. Mystical consciousness can be like that: order, beauty, and meaning, all infinite and multidimensional in scope, that people label "ineffable." Perhaps as more English-speaking people articulate mystical experiences to one another, some new terms may emerge that might prove useful. Greek, for example, has more words than English for love; Sanskrit allegedly has more words to describe and discuss subtle changes in states of meditative awareness.

Another problem in communication with words may be found in the structure of language itself. Our sentences require a subject and a predicate—a temporal sequence. And sometimes in mystical states of consciousness, there is no time. Did "I" have a mystical experience, or did the mystical experience "have me"? The everyday ego or "I" may have experienced its death, yet consciousness of the eternal continued and was recorded in memory before the "I" noticed that it was being reborn into the world of time. That's hard to explain to someone else!

Still another complicating factor in the attempt to communicate these profound states of consciousness is paradox–the manner in which concepts that we consider opposite each other in everyday thought and conversation become encompassed in a reality that includes both extremes. Philosophers call these opposites "antinomies" and ponder them: the one and the many, the universal and the particular, the personal and the nonpersonal, the eternal and the temporal, the male and the female, freedom and determinism, good and evil. From the mountaintop perspective of mystical consciousness, these opposites are often experienced as so meaningfully interrelated that expression demands acknowledgment of "Both/And" rather than "Either/Or." Men and women, striving to articulate their mystical experiences, find themselves saying, "I died, but never felt more alive." Or, "The Void contained All Reality." Or, "The Ultimate Reality I recall was more than a person, yet was suffused with love." Physicists appear to encounter a similar problem when trying to talk about light that is both wave and particle. It is understandable that many people become self-conscious and easily retreat into silence.

So it is that, in being the best wordsmith I can within these pages, I, as well as those whom I have chosen to quote, move fairly freely between scientific and poetic modes of expression.

THE PLACE OF RELIGIOUS EXPERIENCE IN RELIGION

Finally, here are a few introductory words for readers especially interested in the potential relevance of renewed psychedelic research for theology, religious studies, and religious practice. Much of the content of this book centers on primary religious experiences, direct encounters with a sacred dimension of human consciousness that may be viewed as continuing revelation, here and now, in the twenty-first century. It was William James, the Harvard psychologist who published *The Varieties of Religious Experience* in 1902 and who was also known to explore other states of consciousness with the assistance of nitrous oxide gas, who articulated a distinction between primary and secondary religious experiences. *Primary* refers to the experiences that happen directly to you; *secondary* refers to those of others, some of whom have taught you about beliefs, or perhaps have even written down descriptions of their experiential insights that subsequently became enshrined as scripture. Primary forms of religious experience, some perhaps less intense than visionary and mystical states of awareness, may also be understood to include personal devotion, the experiential sense of entrusting one's life to, and perhaps communing with, a sacred dimension greater than one's everyday personality, as is manifested in Bhakti Yoga and many forms of worship and prayer. Precious as such primary states of mind are for those fortunate enough to experience them, regardless of completeness or intensity, I suggest that they constitute but one pillar of what many would consider a balanced and mature religious life.

There are three other pillars, each of which bears its own significance. First, there are sacred scriptures, be they the Torah, the Bible, the Koran, the Vedas, Upanishads and Bhagavad Gita, the Buddhist Sutras, the Sikh Guru Granth Sahib, the Tao Tê Ching, or others. Second, there are theological formulations–basically rational in nature–and unique historical or institutional traditions, changing over time, as found in the Hebrew Talmud, Christian creeds, and the lectures of Shankara (the Advaitan, or nondualist, seer from the eighth century CE) or Ramanuja (a Hindu philosopher who included theistic concepts in the eleventh century CE). Third, there are social expressions of religious belief in compassionate service to others, both within religious congregations or sanghas and in the world at large in the context of Karma Yoga, Buddhist bodhicitta or tonglen, Jewish tzedakah and chesed, Muslim islaah or da'wah, or Sikh langars and Christian hospitals, retirement homes, and soup kitchens. Primary religious experiences may well provide wisdom and vitality that may illumine and strengthen these other religious pillars; however, in my judgment, they do not render them less important. As people vary in their personality structures and styles of being-in-the-world (a good existentialist term), so some may place more weight on one or two of these four pillars than on the others; yet I suggest that all have significance and merit serious study, engagement, and respect.

Manifestations of religion, such as some forms of Gnosticism, that have tended to enthrone direct spiritual experiences and devalue other pillars of the religious enterprise appear to have gradually become cultish, secretive, and ineffective in communicating with those who for whatever reasons are unable to share a common vision. Many people today, perhaps increasing in number, express their dissatisfaction with current institutional forms of religion by describing themselves as "spiritual, but not religious." Some tend to abandon the social expression of spirituality in cohesive religious communities and perhaps unwittingly allow the word "religion" to come to pertain only to the institutional, dogma-centered manifestations that they may view as lacking in inspiration, vitality, and relevance in the modern scientific world.

If indeed the word "religion," originating in the Latin *religare*, is to continue to signify that which most profoundly binds us together and reflects a shared perspective on what gives life its deepest purpose and meaning, I personally do not support abandoning it in favor of "spirituality." Throughout the ages, most religious institutions have respectfully included and accommodated experiences called spiritual or religious, however engendered. The Constitution of the United States of America protects "freedom of religion"; nothing is said about "freedom of spirituality." It is my hope that the leaders of religious institutions in each of the world religions will become emboldened to thoughtfully accommodate the potential contributions of entheogens in good time, as their styles of theological thinking and religious practices continue to evolve in order to more firmly connect with the spiritual yearnings and intellectual understandings of those they are dedicated to serving. If and when entheogens become legally available as elective tools in theological education and in religious retreats and practices, I trust that the experiences they occasion will contribute to balanced religious lives and healthy religious communities.

3

Revelation and Doubt

INITIAL COGNITIVE ADJUSTMENTS

What does one do with a mystical experience? Or, perhaps better expressed, what does a mystical experience do with you? Following that first encounter with mystical states of consciousness, as described in the preface, I became known in the psychiatric clinic in Göttingen as "that American student who had the interesting mystical experience." My experiential report was atypical at the time, since relatively low dosage was being administered with little preparation or emotional support and with essentially no knowledge of how to maximize safety and potential benefit. Other volunteers had tended to experience sensory and perceptual changes, memories from early childhood, and occasionally episodes of anxiety, physical discomfort, or paranoid thought processes.

Whether I may have been a "natural mystic" on the verge of encountering this profound form of consciousness spontaneously, and thus required only a low dose of psilocybin to facilitate the experience, or whether I was experiencing sufficient stress and insecurity (having just arrived, alone in a new country, immersed in a new language) to trigger such phenomena, I will never know. I had always experienced a mild awareness of a sacred dimension, especially as manifested in the pristine beauty of the rugged and fragrant pine forests on the shores of Lake Superior where I grew up in the Upper Peninsula of Michigan, but nothing of this magnitude. At the time, I was not at all sure that "I" had the experience; it seemed equally valid to say that the experience "had me." The best way I could express it in language was to say that the memory of it remained vividly accessible in my awareness as I sat in university classrooms and walked the streets of the everyday world. In truth, it proved to be a pivotal fulcrum that provided clarity and direction as my subsequent path in life gradually unfolded before me.

The research design of the study in which I had participated entailed the administration of either of two shorter-acting derivatives of psilocybin (facilitating around four hours of alternative states instead of the usual six), designated as CEY-19 and CZ-74. For readers who understand something of the language of chemistry, psilocybin, historically designated as C-39 (4-phosphoryloxy-N,N-dimethyltryptamine), after ingestion is converted into psilocin (4-hydroxy-N,N-dimethyltryptamine) by biochemical processes in the body. Like psilocybin, CEY-19 (4-phosphoryloxy-N,N-diethyltryptamine) after ingestion is also converted in the body into CZ-74 (4-hydroxy-N,N-diethyltryptamine), which is the active compound. Administered at four weekly intervals, this investigation intended to blindly compare the effects of the two shorter-acting substances. I later learned that my initial experience was occasioned by 13 mg of CZ-74; in the next three research sessions I received injections of 13 mg of CEY-19, 16 mg of CEY-19, and 16 mg of CZ-74.

With a mixture of hope and trepidation, I anticipated a reoccurrence of mystical phenomena on each of those three subsequent occasions, but none manifested themselves. I experienced deep relaxation and minor sensory changes, accompanied by some philosophical rumination that may have been insightful, but nothing that I could consider of real revelatory or religious import. When I wrote in my journal following the fourth and final experiment in this series, I was troubled and wondered if I had been naïve and gullible, if I had exaggerated whatever occurred in that first experience. Maybe what I had called mystical consciousness really simply had been sensual pleasure of some kind. The pendulum of my theological orientation was starting to shift away from the experiential theories of the religious existential-ists to the conservative styles of thinking then called neo-orthodox. At the very least, it was obvious that more was involved in facilitating mystical forms of experience than simply receiving an entheogen and experiencing a "drug effect."

THE CONTRIBUTIONS OF WALTER PAHNKE

At that juncture, Walter Norman Pahnke arrived in Göttingen on a traveling fellowship from Harvard University, along with his wife Eva and their daughter Kristin, a young, blonde toddler. We met in Leun-er's clinic and rapidly became good friends. Now visiting centers in Europe where research with psychedelic substances was taking place, Wally (with his doctor of medicine, master of divinity, and psychiatric residency, all from Harvard, behind him) had conducted the research project known as the "Good Friday Experiment" for his PhD disserta-tion in the History and Philosophy of Religion on the subject of Reli-gion and Society. To demonstrate with double-blind methods that psi-locybin indeed could occasion mystical experiences that were similar, if not identical, to those recorded in the literature of mysticism, he had administered either 30 mg of psilocybin or 200 mg of niacin (Vitamin B-3, also known as nicotinic acid, which briefly causes mild dizziness and tingling sensations) in capsules identical in appearance.

His volunteer subjects were twenty theological students from the nearby Andover-Newton Theological School and ten professors or graduate students from nearby universities who served as guides. Two guides were assigned to each of five subgroups of four theological stu-dents, and one guide in each pair was randomly designated to receive psilocybin and the other niacin. All expected an inactive placebo to be used in the study, so suggestion was maximized for those who received the niacin. The experiment was conducted in a small worship space in the undercroft of Boston University's Marsh Chapel. Concur-rently, the annual Good Friday Service, presided over by the eminent African American preacher Howard Thurman (himself, a man with mystical sensitivities), was taking place in the main sanctuary upstairs and was transmitted through loudspeakers into the basement chapel. This occurred on April 20, 1962, and became known through press coverage as "the Miracle in Marsh Chapel." Wally's hypothesis was well supported by the data, which had consisted of questionnaires and interviews.

Now, in February 1964, Wally, in spite of his intense interest and curiosity, had still never taken a psychedelic substance himself and, not without uncertainty and anxiety, patiently was awaiting confirmation of the award of his PhD degree. Controversy was surrounding psychedelic drugs at Harvard, and two of his academic supporters, Timothy Leary and Richard Alpert (subsequently known as Ram Dass), had been dismissed by the university in the spring of 1963–Leary first for leaving town and his teaching responsibilities without proper notice, and then Alpert for giving psilocybin to an undergraduate student after agreeing to limit his research volunteers to graduate students only.

Hearing the story of my history as a research participant and my current perplexity about the significance of it all, Wally rather impishly proposed a fifth drug administration to Dr. Leuner. What might happen if Bill Richards were given a slightly larger dose of psilocybin? He also suggested that the experimental session be conducted in a room of the clinic on the second floor with more light, plus some plants and music, and that he stay with me to offer emotional support if needed. I was open to the idea and Dr. Leuner was happy to approve the plan. So Wally and I went shopping for music, which included a 33-rpm recording of the Brahms's German Requiem and a 45-rpm issue of J. S. Bach's Fantasia and Fugue in G Minor for pipe organ. So it was that, on Valentine's Day in 1964, I received an intramuscular injection of 28 mg of CEY-19.

SESSION NUMBER FIVE AND ITS AFTEREFFECTS

Relatively soon after psilocybin administration, the mystical forms of consciousness recurred in all their splendor, repeatedly drawing my being through several cycles of psychological death and rebirth, the noetic intensity of spiritual knowledge feeling etched into my brain. In the research report I subsequently wrote, there were terms such as "cosmic tenderness," "infinite love," "penetrating peace," "eternal blessing," and "unconditional acceptance," coupled with "unspeakable awe," "overflowing joy," "primeval humility," "inexpressible gratitude," and "boundless devotion," all followed by the sentence, "Yet all of these words are hopelessly inadequate and can do little more than meekly point toward the genuine, inexpressible feelings actually experienced." I had not exaggerated what had occurred in that first experience; I felt as though I had forgotten 80 percent of it. Never since that time have I personally doubted the reality and validity of this state of awareness, and now over fifty years have passed. On rare occasions, with the help of meditative disciplines, while immersed in the natural world, in the midst of personal musical performance, or with the assistance of psychedelic substances, this clarity of awareness has been refreshed and nurtured.

In lectures and professional publications over the years, I have discussed different ways of interpreting such profound human experiences. One could choose to employ labels like "cognitive impairment," "wishful thinking," "hypomanic episode," or "regression to infantile functioning," or posit that mystical consciousness might merely be a convincing delusion and defense mechanism in the face of death. There are rational arguments to defuse each suggestion that might question or devalue the import of such revelatory states of mind, above all calling attention to the repetition of very similar descriptions throughout history in different cultures and the ethical imperatives, creative insights, and courageous leadership that have often been manifested in their wake. Ultimately, however, I have come to view it as a matter of personal choice to affirm experiential, intuitive knowledge. In that respect, believing in the validity of mystical consciousness is similar to believing that one truly loves one's spouse or children. One lives out of such convictions. The memory of mystical consciousness, for better or worse, structures my Weltanschauung, or view of the world. As succinctly expressed by the anthropologist Jeremy Narby in the documentary film *Neurons to Nirvana*, in reference to his own personal experience during the effects of ayahuasca, "Once you drink you see, and once you see you can't unsee."

In Walter Pahnke's definition of the term "mystical consciousness," he included a category titled "Persisting Positive Changes in Attitudes and Behavior." Although not intrinsic to the immediate, experiential content of this alternate state of consciousness, this category is often considered when debating the alleged validity of mystical experiences reported throughout history, however they may have been engendered. Huston Smith, an eminent scholar of comparative religions, articulated this well in his distinction between "religious experiences" and "religious lives" and also between "states of consciousness" and "traits of behavior." A mark of true spirituality in Buddhism is the humble return of the awakening adept from the summit of enlightenment to a life of service in the marketplace where the need for compassion is greatest. In the Jewish-Christian heritage, the model of Deutero-Isaiah is germane, focusing on the "Suffering Servant" as the true emissary of Yahweh. Perhaps this is where Timothy Leary, or at least the popular interpretation of his words, went awry: instead of "turn on, tune in, and drop out," the message should have been "turn on, tune in, and jump in." The emphasis could have been placed on expressing caring for others and the world by respectfully engaging those who may tend to have different perspectives or values while working diligently to implement one's visionary insights in and through existing social structures.

Over the years, as I have observed the changes in attitudes and behavior manifested by research volunteers in the wake of mystical consciousness, this factor has proved to be of fundamental significance. In the classical literature of mysticism, the first visionary or mystical experience is often understood to signal the Awakening or beginning of spiritual development, to be followed by Purgation, often including what St. John of the Cross back in the sixteenth century called "The Dark Night of the Soul." Then gradual Illumination unfolds with eventual glimpses of a return to unitive consciousness, coupled with becoming an increasingly compassionate presence in the everyday world.

Clearly the first epiphany is no confirmation of sainthood. It might be viewed as a helicopter ride to the glorious peak of the spiritual mountain, but when one returns to camp at the base with the challenging path winding upward through difficult terrain, the climbing still needs to be done. Yet many appear to then become motivated to climb as never before. Now, there is no question that there really is a summit to the mountain, that the perspective from that pinnacle is worth all the effort and anguish of the spiritual journey, and that the journey itself has meaning. Many who are now committed to disciplined meditative practices and compassionate action, some of whom might well decline an opportunity to receive an entheogen even if it were legally accessible, will also acknowledge that their interest in spiritual development was originally awakened or significantly nurtured by an experience occasioned by a psychedelic substance.

In my own personal journaling at age twenty-three, I found in the aftermath of mystical consciousness what I considered a healthy independence from social pressures and increased freedom to authentically "be myself." In accordance with existential theory, I felt less like a puppet controlled by the social expectations that impinged on my life. With this shift there came a sense of inner peace, increased self-confidence, and a notable decrease in anxiety. I think I also became less inhibited, more spontaneous, perhaps more playful, and more capable of allowing relationships characterized by genuineness and intimacy to develop. I felt attuned to "what really mattered," at least for me at that stage of my life. Paul Tillich's term for this was "the courage to be," including "the courage to accept acceptance." Coupled with the intuitive insights discussed in the following chapter, I think those who know me well would say that, since that time, I have tended to maintain a sense of centeredness and deep optimism, even amid major stressors and life changes, including the death of my wife and, not insignificantly, the transition in employment and professional identity in 1977 when the psychedelic research to which I had so deeply dedicated myself was rendered dormant in the United States. At that point, I attempted to personally apply the mantram we often gave our research volunteers to help guide them through difficult transitions in consciousness: Trust, Let go, and Be open.

Thus, I have chosen to trust the validity of the memories of visionary and mystical forms of consciousness that are still accessible in my field of mental awareness in everyday life. Each reader who has encountered similar experiences, with or without the use of entheogens, must similarly weigh possible revelation and doubt and make his or her own inner judgments. Undeniably, there are mild experiences that some recall that may well have been induced by suggestion and imagination. Further, there is a middle ground where experiences of aesthetic enhancement and abstract imagery begin to merge into terrain of more potent spiritual knowledge. Imagination, after all, is the mind creatively producing images, and some of those images may be rich in meaning and personal truth, relevant to everyday living or to spiritual knowledge. My own resolution of this issue is to honor and respect most any experience that another person treasures as sacred. The one exception to this guideline would be if and when someone felt compelled to act in the world in a manner I considered blatantly irrational or destructive, citing an alleged revelatory state of consciousness as the justification for such behavior. Here reason and the combined revelatory experiences of others would be summoned in the process of making the wisest possible judgment. In my experience, the spiritual insights treasured by most people who have known mystical forms of experience are remarkably similar.

PART II

Mystical and Visionary Forms of Consciousness

4

Intuitive Knowledge

One reason the study of mystical forms of consciousness is of importance is that the experiences entail more than emotion–however exalted and elevated the feelings may be. Such experiences, both in the mystical literature of each world religion and in modern psychedelic research, are also claimed to include knowledge. Often there are descriptions of "beholding truth." William James, the Harvard psychologist who published *The Varieties of Religious Experience* in 1902, chose to call this "the noetic quality" of mystical experiences. More recently, in *Mysticism and Philosophy*, published in 1960, Walter T. Stace from Princeton University formulated the category "Objectivity and Reality" to account not only for the certainty of intuitive knowledge, but also for the convincing intensity of such states of awareness.

Sigmund Freud, in spite of his many creative contributions to helping us understand the workings of our minds, was one person who had trouble comprehending this aspect of mental functioning. He called it "the oceanic feeling." This term for mystical consciousness had been coined by Romain Rolland, a Frenchman who was a novelist, poet, and mystic and who, Freud wrote in his book *Civilization and Its Discontents*, "calls himself my friend." Unable to find mystical consciousness within his own mind, Freud himself tended to devalue the import of the experience and chose to interpret it as a memory of union with the mother's breast before the individual self or ego developed. Yet even he acknowledged that "there may be something else behind this, but for the present it is wrapped in obscurity."

If the experience is understood as regression, even regression beyond the breast to memories of life in the womb, it appears that there is much more going on within the womb than Freud ever imagined. From the viewpoint of those who have known mystical forms of consciousness, the approach through changes in time perception to eternal dimensions may be understood either as regression or as progression, and the content discovered is usually described as substantially more than feelings alone. The poet William Wordsworth in his *Ode on Intimations of Immortality from Recollections of Early Childhood* may have been more on target, writing that "trailing clouds of glory do we come / From God, who is our home: / Heaven lies about us in our infancy!"

We tend to think of experiential domains as "subjective," of intuition at best as "a woman's hunch," and have learned to think of objective knowledge as inevitably associated with the cognitive process we call "thinking" or "reason." In contrast, scholars of mysticism take intuitive knowledge seriously and point to two ways of knowing: intuition and rational thought. Rudolf Otto, the German theologian and scholar of comparative religions who in 1917 published *Das Heilige* (translated as *The Idea of the Holy*), formulated three categories of human mental processes: (1) the rational, (2) the irrational, and (3) the nonrational. It is his third category that accommodates the claims of the mystics.

When we reflect rationally on mystical literature or on the research reports of volunteers who have received psychedelic substances, how can we tell what may be "irrational" and what may be "nonrational"? Although this question can endlessly delight philosophers who specialize in epistemology, the mental gymnastics of trying to articulate and defend how we know what we think we know, it may be useful to examine two simple perspectives: (1) how the intuitive knowledge that one person reports compares to what others have reported, and (2) the subsequent attitudes and behavior manifested in the wake of the alleged knowledge, which William James called the "fruits for life."

To address the first perspective, let it be noted that there are several tenets of knowledge that tend to be reported and "hang together" following mystical forms of experience. With acknowledgment of the limitations of language and how different words vary in meaning for different people, I will simply list and briefly discuss several of these tenets. The common core of insights typically includes the reality of (1) God, (2) immortality, (3) interrelationships, (4) love, (5) beauty, and (6) emerging wisdom.

GOD

This simple three-letter word (in English) has many variations of meaning for different people and evokes passions ranging from total devotion and awe to total indifference and disgust. For some, it conjures up an image of Michelangelo's creator God on the ceiling of the Sistine Chapel in Rome, a rather heavy-set man with a bushy white beard, surrounded by cherubs, dressed in a translucent garment, somewhere up there in the clouds, perhaps dodging jet planes. If he exists, he appears to be quite irrelevant to those who struggle through daily life. For others, God may be a destructive force, perhaps judgmental, manifested in thunder, plagues, earthquakes, tsunamis, and fatal illnesses. I have learned over the years that, when people label themselves as atheists and I ask what sort of God they don't believe in, I often end up agreeing with them. Often, their concepts of God are quite undeveloped and still shaded by rebellion against ideas that adults, it is hoped well meaning, tried to force upon them in childhood and adolescence. Some immediately recall trying not to wiggle in uncomfortable pews during long, boring sermons. Others have experienced painful losses or life traumas that still eclipse their attempts to find meaning in any of the religious frameworks that they have encountered. Many have never had the opportunity or have never taken the time to explore concepts of God more in harmony with the perspectives of mystics and scholars on frontiers of science.

A fascinating discovery in speaking with mystics from different world religions is how secure they appear in their certainty of the reality of a sacred dimension of consciousness and how little they care about what words one may choose to describe it. If you like the word "God," that's fine; if you prefer "Yahweh," "Jehovah," "The Christ Consciousness," "Allah," "Brahman," "The Great Spirit," or simply "The

Higher Power," that's also OK. If you would rather verbalize the ultimate reality as "The Void," "Nothingness," "Nondual Awareness," "The Pure Land," or "Celestial Buddha Fields," even that is acceptable. Many words have been used in different religious traditions and philosophical systems, such as Rudolf Otto's "Numinous," Paul Tillich's "The Ground of Being," and even the Yale biologist Edmund Sinnott's "the purposive properties of protoplasm." Some Star Wars aficionados may be content simply to say, "May the Force be with you." A theologian we have called Pseudo-Dionysius the Areopagite, one credited with interrelating Neo-Platonic and early Christian thought in the late fifth century or early sixth, was fond of the term "The Nameless."

Wayne Teasdale, both a Christian and a Buddhist monk who personally understood mystical consciousness and the promise of entheogens when wisely ingested, coined the term "interspirituality" to depict a mountain of truth with a common summit but many paths leading from its base to its ineffable peak. Within this model, each path is worth traveling and contains its own unique historical traditions and symbolic expressions of spiritual truths—its own wisdom and inspiration. Since no one person can travel all the paths at the same time, it generally makes sense to embrace the tradition of one's childhood or culture, to learn to speak that language and appreciate the stories and ritual expressions that go with it. Yet one can travel on one's own path and still respect and appreciate the paths of others that may be different. One can proudly own one's own heritage and share it with one's children as a valued treasure and still remain open to learning from other traditions, taking delight in finding common ground and in sharing differences in perspectives.

Within this metaphor, the paths come closer to one another as the summit of the mountain is approached. So it is that it becomes possible for a Christian to worship genuinely in a Hindu temple, a Jew to bow to Allah in an Islamic Mosque, a Buddhist to recite a Taoist prayer, or any other combination. Scriptures come to mind: "Hear, O Israel, the Lord our God is One" (Deut. 6:4). "Before Abraham was, I am" (John 8:58). "Say (Muhammad): He is God, the One and Only; God, the Eternal, Absolute; He begetteth not, nor is He begotten; And there is none like unto Him" (Qur'an 112:1–4). "There is only one God, not the second; not at all, not at all, not in the least bit" (the Brahma

Sutra). Those whose childhood experiences included singing around campfires at church or scout camps may well recall the song "He's Got the Whole Wide World in His Hands." It appears that the greater the awareness of the eternal grows in human consciousness, the less preoccupied the everyday personality becomes with its own favorite collection of words and concepts.

Before some religious scholars become critically disparaging or dismissive in response to the prior paragraph, let me again invoke the principles of ineffability and paradoxicality and request that readers attempt at least temporarily to suspend those words and concepts that structure our usual lives, be they religious or nonreligious. This is important because the experiential knowledge of "One God," as will subsequently be discussed, also brings with it, if taken seriously, an awareness of the interconnectedness and interrelationships of all peoples irrespective of their national or cultural origins, which, in turn, has profound implications for intercultural understanding, ethics, and world peace. No matter how rich and personally meaningful our own religious heritages and practices may be, in the world of the twenty-first century it is myopically dangerous to ignore or devalue the traditions and perspectives of other cultures.

In approaching respectful understanding of the diversity of religious languages and traditions, it is also of critical importance to comprehend that there is a variety of very meaningful religious experiences. At this point in our discussion, the spotlight is on mystical consciousness, defined as a unitive awareness. Here, in the language of Hinduism, the Atman of the individual self recognizes that it is an integral fragment of the universal Brahman, as a single drop of water may fall into the vast ocean and merge with it. This is undeniably one form of experience reported in the historic literature of mysticism and by volunteers in projects of psychedelic research, and the profundity of the memory is almost unspeakably meaningful.

Yet this does not preclude other varieties of religious experience, such as visionary forms of awareness in which the everyday self relates lovingly with the divine, or states of conversion when guilt and grief are transformed by convincing feelings of forgiveness and unconditional acceptance, or the simple, quiet feelings of the presence of the divine in periods of prayer, meditation, serene love making, or communion with nature. All of these potential experiences, and undoubtedly even others, appear to be part of the human repertoire and may well be accessible to most, if not all, people. In subsequent chapters, these other states of mind will receive more attention.

Especially in Western religions, we have been very wary when speaking of the relationship between God (that is, ultimate reality) and human beings (that is, homo sapiens, or what theologians historically have called "Man"). Hebrew and Christian theology, along with some Islamic sources, includes the concept of the *imago dei*, the "image" of God in which we were created, and different theologians have debated whether the image denotes shared essence or merely a mirrored reflection. Quakers acknowledge the "inner light," a spark of divine energy implanted like a seed within us all that may sprout into firsthand religious experiences. A similar perspective is found in the writings of Inayat Kahn, an Islamic Sufi, who discussed "Man, the Seed of God." John Wesley, the founder of Methodism, interpreted his experience of his heart being "strangely warmed" as the presence of Christ, a manifestation of God in his life, and many Protestant evangelical denominations have continued to deeply respect and attempt to facilitate such experiences of religious conversion. In monastic communities, Eastern Orthodox, Roman Catholic, Episcopal, and Buddhist, experiences deemed revelatory or sacred tend to be deeply valued, though they may be verbally expressed in different ways.

So it is that Western preconceptions and language are poorly prepared to come to terms with the experience of the Atman/Brahman Unity as expressed in Hinduism. When a Western person says, "I am God," even if as a poetic utterance, our impulse is to interpret the statement as a psychotic inflation of the ego and to urgently provide psychiatric counsel, if not inpatient hospitalization and antipsychotic medications. As mental health practitioners know well, there indeed are persons who make such claims who are also disoriented, confused, and unable to responsibly care for themselves and function safely in the world. For these people, hospitalization may be required to ensure safety and provide new grounding and reorientation in life.

It might help, however, if more mental health professionals appreciated that some of these people may be expressing a glimpse of a very impressive and potentially meaningful state of consciousness that they are presently unable to successfully integrate into their everyday lives, rather than simply dismissing their claims as "crazy." A reasonably well-integrated, stable person with articulate verbal skills who recalls such a profound unitive state of consciousness, were he to speak at all, might own the ultimate insight that in the final analysis the energy that makes up his life is "God," but this would be without inflation of the ego, since he also would acknowledge that the same is true of every other human being. Philosophers call this perspective *panentheism*, not simply that "everything is God" (that is, *pantheism*), but rather that the Sacred is to be found in the ultimate source or core of being. The Hindu tradition of 330 million deities, all of whom may be understood as facets of one unspeakably magnificent diamond of spiritual truth, or one ultimate Brahman, may also prove helpful in coping with the paradox of the relationship between ourselves and God or whatever term we may personally choose to point toward Ultimate Reality.

As illustration, let us consider two quotations from the personal reports of an eminent scholar of world religions, Huston Smith: the first, a classical Hindu experience, facilitated by mescaline; the second, a personal, more traditional Christian experience, which happened to be occasioned by psilocybin when he was serving as a guide during Walter Pahnke's Good Friday Experiment. Both quotations have been published in other sources in the past, including Smith's book *Cleansing the Doors of Perception*.

> The world into which I was ushered was strange, weird, uncanny, significant, and terrifying beyond belief. . . . Plotinus's emanation theory, and its more detailed Vedantic counterpart, had hitherto been only conceptual theories for me. Now I was *seeing* them, with their descending bands spread out before me. I found myself amused, thinking how duped historians of philosophy had been in crediting the originators of such worldviews with being specu-lative geniuses. Had they had experiences such as mine, they need have been no more than hack reporters. But beyond accounting for the origin of these philosophies, my experience supported their truth. As in Plato's myth of the cave, what I was now seeing struck me with the force of the sun, in comparison with which everyday experience reveals only flickering shadows in a dim

cavern. How could these layers upon layers, these worlds within worlds, these paradoxes in which I could be both myself *and* my world and an episode be both momentary *and* eternal–how could such things be put into words?

The experiment was powerful for me, and it left a permanent mark on my experienced worldview. (I say "experienced worldview" to distinguish it from what I think and believe the world is like.) For as long as I can remember I have believed in God, and I experienced his presence both within the world and when the world was transcendentally eclipsed. But until the Good Friday Experiment, I had had no direct personal encounter with God of the sort that *bhakti yogis*, Pentecostals, and born-again Christians describe. The Good Friday Experiment changed that, presumably because the service focused on God as incarnate in Christ. . . . For me, the climax of the service came during a solo that was sung by a soprano whose voice (as it came to me through the prism of psilocybin) I can only describe as angelic. What she sang was no more than a simple hymn, but it entered my soul so deeply that its opening and closing verses have stayed with me ever since . . . *My times are in Thy hands, my God* . . . the gestalt transformed a routine musical progression into the most powerful cosmic homecoming I have ever experienced.

IMMORTALITY

During mystical experiences, there is often an intuitive conviction that the eternal realms of consciousness are indestructible and not subject to time. This insight is typically reported as having been blatantly obvious when mystical consciousness was occurring. "Consciousness" from this perspective perhaps may be best understood as the ultimate energy that makes up all that is and is to be found at the core of all that is. Such energy may change form or evolve–or dance as depicted in the Hindu image of Nataraja, the dancing Shiva–but it cannot cease to be. Paradoxically, it may simultaneously be experienced both as the unchanging One described by the ancient Greek philosopher Parmenides and as the constantly changing river of life emphasized by his compatriot,

Heraclitus. This understanding of the ultimate nature of energy is, as many readers may realize, similar to the views of quantum physicists. As noted in books like Fritjof Capra's *The Tao of Physics*, the writings of mystics and physicists often sound very similar. The religious word for this indestructibility of energy is "immortality"; the mathematical word is "infinity." In philosophical circles this may be called "panpsychism," a way of viewing reality in which everything is ultimately understood to be the energy some of us would call mind or consciousness.

This intuitive insight within mystical consciousness is especially relevant for those of us who are mortal, and especially for people in close proximity of the experience we call "death." One of the most meaningful aspects of my career in psychedelic research has entailed administering entheogens to terminal cancer patients in the context of brief psychotherapy and supporting them through various alternative states of human consciousness. When mystical forms of experience have occurred, there has almost always been reported a concomitant loss of the fear of death, which, in turn, contributes to reduced depression, anxiety, preoccupation with pain, and interpersonal isolation, and often enables the person with cancer to live the remainder of his or her current lifetime more fully. Research in this humane application of psychedelics in medicine is once again in process, with recent studies at the University of California in Los Angeles, at the Johns Hopkins School of Medicine, at New York University, and in Solothurn, Switzerland, perhaps paving the way for the legal offering of an intervention, most likely with psilocybin, to appropriate people in palliative care divisions of hospitals and in hospices in the foreseeable future.

In illustration, consider this report, written by a thirty-one-year-old cancer patient, married with two children and suffering from advancing Stage IV lymphoma, who received the psychedelic substance dipropyltryptamine (DPT):

[After entheogen administration] I first went to a place that seemed to completely lack the qualities of this world as we know it. I seemed to transcend time and space and I lost complete identification with the "real" world. The experience seemed to me to be as if I was going from this world back to another world before this life had occurred. . . . The actual changing from this life to whatever was before this life seemed to be involved in a very bright silver mass of energy with very strong electrical current. . . . Strangely enough I felt that I had been in that mass of energy at one time before. When I was there everything seemed to make sense. . . . It was a very beautiful world, one in which love was very much a part. . . . The basic theme that I perceived . . . was that life continues to go on and we are basically some form of essence from a Supreme Being and we are part of that Supreme Being. . . . I don't have the fear of death that I once had. . . . I have found that everyday living seems to be much more enjoyable. Small things in life that I may have overlooked I seem to appreciate now. I have a much greater and deeper understanding of other people . . . and a much greater capacity to try to fulfill other people's needs. . . . Overall I think that I am a much more content individual, having had the great opportunity to just glimpse for a very short moment the overall thinking of God, of possibly being brought into His confidence for just a brief period, to be reassured that there is a very beautiful, loving masterful plan in this Universe for all of us.

It is of interest that cancer patients and others who find such profound mystical experiences in their memory banks are not necessarily convinced of personal immortality, that is, the continued existence after death of the everyday personality that goes with our common names. "Life *after* death" implies a temporal sequence. Rather, they tend to report a conviction that Eternity, or Infinity, a state of consciousness outside of time, is so unquestionably real to them that it does not matter one way or another whether the everyday personality survives when the body stops functioning and decomposes. They often express a conviction that ultimately "all is well" in the universe, reminiscent of the familiar words of the fourteenth-century English mystic Julian of Norwich, who is known for saying, "All shall be well, and all shall be well, and all manner of thing shall be well." One volunteer wrote, "I know that Being is eternal, whether I exist or not. I have no fear of losing my ego." This could be understood in the framework of Zen Buddhism, in which it is believed that, if one can be fully present, one can find in the center of each moment a portal that opens to the Infinite. The spiritual world thus not only may be seen as awaiting us before time (birth) and after time (death), but also is always to be found in the "Eternal Now," with or without a functioning body. In Christian language, it may be described as awakening to the "Christ conscious-ness" or "resting in the arms of the Lord."

These reports from the perspective of unitive-mystical conscious-ness of course do not rule out the possibility of personal immortality. There are other states of consciousness that may well be relevant to understanding death from other perspectives. I recall a research volun-teer who was convinced that he had spent approximately two hours during his psilocybin session in a meaningful and personally helpful conversation with his deceased brother. Similarly, it is not uncommon to feel immersed in another historical period or life-story, which some interpret as evidence for reincarnation. Whether indicative of the cre-ative acumen of a novelist or literal experiences within unique states of consciousness, such reports merit respect while we may withhold judgment about their ontological validity.

INTERRELATIONSHIPS

Logically, it makes sense that if, indeed, there is a great unity or one-ness, that every part of that unity must somehow be interconnected and interrelated. From the experiential perspective of mystical con-sciousness, this is often avowed to be literally true. On the human level, every person is a member of the "family of man," your own brother or sister, all of whom may be understood as emanations from the univer-sal source, quite in harmony with the Neo-Platonic theory of Plotinus, a Greek philosopher who lived in the early second century CE, and of course with Plato himself before him. It is intriguing to speculate on Plato's participation in the Eleusinian mystery religions that included the ritual ingestion of a hallucinogenic brew called *kykeon* and how his ideas might have been influenced by his own entheogenic expe-riences. In the symbolic language of Hinduism, this interconnected-ness may be understood as part of the bejeweled web or net of Indra, the Vedic Lord of Heaven, in which we all participate. As the English language has accommodated the women's movement, the time has come to leave terms with masculine bias like "mankind" and "family of man" in the dust of history and refer to "humankind" and "the human family" instead.

If we humans are indeed all relatives, linked both through our genes and in the spiritual vortices of our minds, we must also acknowledge the emphasis that existential philosophers have placed on struggle as an intrinsic part of human existence. We do tend to fight with one another in the realm of ideas debated in universities, in the chambers of the United Nations, and sometimes on actual battlefields. Sometimes the struggle is akin to two friends arm wrestling in good-natured style; sometimes it becomes the ugly devaluing of the other and the urge to destroy the other. How we cope with anger and our definitions of "good" and "evil" become prominent here and we act out our parts with passion on the ever-changing stage of human history.

In the cosmic dance of Shiva, individual lives, civilizations, and even solar systems and galaxies are understood to come into being and go out of being. They are created and then destroyed, not unlike when a child builds a tower with blocks, gleefully knocks it over, and then builds once again. From this perspective, the processes of death and rebirth, of all we consider dreadful and all we view as glorious, are integral to the nature of ultimate reality. God dances in the creative process that always continues, sometimes fiercely and majestically, sometimes joyfully and playfully. The image of the Hindu god Kali depicts this well: a dark mother goddess with human skulls hanging around her neck whose image may be found hanging on the walls of many Indian living rooms, not as a threat to be feared, but as a manifestation of the divine to be loved.

An experience in South America occasioned by ayahuasca comes to mind, the description of which was titled "The Garden of Souls." Within it every human being was a unique work of art in the process of creation, all together on an infinite chessboard. Philosophical concepts of freedom and determinism come into play here. None of us creates ourselves, yet through the gift of freedom we participate in the uniqueness of our individual lives. Philosophers and theologians reflect on this gift of freedom, without which we would be robots, and on the challenge to use the gift wisely. Perhaps there are times when the divine intelligence at the core of being (for those who can imagine such a construct) compassionately views the messes we humans have created, in our wars, our environmental degradation, and our social injustices. Yet, while bemoaning the slowness of our evolution and awakening, one could imagine that the Divine still affirms faith in the primal decision to have endowed us with the freedom to think and choose. Philosophers of history may see a gradual evolution in process as time progresses toward "the Kingdom of God" or some future Utopia. Teilhard de Chardin, for example, saw us gradually progressing, sometimes kicking and screaming, toward "the Omega Point" when consciousness and the universe will "become one."

LOVE

At the conclusion of *The Divine Comedy*, Dante Alighieri, perhaps writing out of his own mystical experiences, concluded, "It is love that moves the sun and other stars" (*Paradiso* 33:145). In mystical consciousness, this love is typically known and subsequently described as much more than human emotion. Poetic and idealistic as it sounds, it is often claimed to be the ultimate nature of the energy that makes up the world, awaiting us all in the source or ground of our being. One cannot help but note that Dante chose the word "comedy" to embrace all the dramas of hell, purgatory, and heaven in his book, perhaps congruent with the Hindu concept of *lila* or divine play. In spite of all the pathos and tragedies we experience in daily temporal existence, mystics testify to the validity of a transcendental perspective beyond usual human cognition where all makes sense in an eternal world permeated by love.

As emphasized by theologians like the Protestant scholar Edgar Sheffield Brightman, love may often be understood as a manifestation of the personal nature of God. A loving relationship between an individual person and God does constitute a devotional baseline in much of Christianity and in Bhakti Yoga. Many of us daily direct inner cascades of words, formal or spontaneous, called prayer to Lord Jehovah, Lord Jesus, Lord Krishna, or Lord Buddha, entrusting "all that one is" to "the Lord." Mystics through the ages, typified by St. Teresa of Avila, have especially exemplified this form of experience. Formalized styles of prayer, notably in Judaism and Islam, and often in Christianity, may or may not entail this personal, experiential feeling of being in relationship with something or someone sacred. Friedrich Heiler, a German theologian who wrote a book called *Das Gebet* (Prayer) back in 1932, suggested simply that prayer is what we discover ourselves doing when life gets sufficiently difficult, whether we believe in any particular religious framework or not. In this perspective, prayer may be seen as a basic human instinct to seek for a spiritual connection with something beyond the everyday personality.

Though it sometimes may be more a matter of language than actual experience, more abstract and universal ways of experiencing and expressing this ultimate love often occur in the reports of those who have known mystical consciousness. God may be described as "more than a person." Thus, as illustrated in the earlier quotations from Huston Smith, there appear to be two ways to encounter this ultimate energy: one in relationship between the everyday self and God, and one in the ineffable merging of identities–another instance of paradoxicality, the Both/And principle. Again, it is not a question of "which is right"; rather, there appear to be two different ways (if not more) in which love may be discovered and experienced in alternative states of awareness. On different occasions, it appears that the same person can experience both forms of consciousness or that one may open into the other.

BEAUTY

Another tenet of the intuitive knowledge often reported in the wake of mystical states of awareness concerns what some would call the absoluteness of beauty. This is a rather radical claim for us in a culture that tends to view little as "absolute," especially when it comes to judgments of art. We like to say, "Beauty is in the eye of the beholder." From the perspective of mystical consciousness, it may be not only "in the eye," but also in the brain and in the mind (whatever that ultimately may be understood to be).

During the action of entheogens in sufficient dosage, most people report a sense of awe at how much they can see with their eyes closed. Eyes suddenly, as in dreaming, seem to have little if anything to do with seeing. The intricate visionary patterns often discovered, sometimes of abstract lines, often initially of pure gold on a jet-black background, reminiscent of the vaulting of Gothic cathedrals, intricately decorated Romanesque arches, or the symmetrically unfolding designs in the domes of some Islamic mosques, tend to evoke feelings of amazement. Then, as if entering the Platonic world of Forms, one may encounter exquisite, richly colored, and detailed images of gods and goddesses, precious gemstones and metals, living sculptures of museum quality, vast landscapes, stretches of outer space, and so forth. Where does all this come from? Is this heaven, God's "dwelling place"? Typically one does not "think" that these images are beautiful, as if one were making a value judgment; rather, one intuitively recognizes them as beautiful and may seem to dissolve into them and participate in the magnificence portrayed. The pure quantity of such imagery is often striking. One person described the rapid flow of images as "roller-skating through the Louvre," occasionally pausing to ponder a single masterpiece and the revelations it contains and then zooming down corridors containing countless paintings and sculptures, all of incredible beauty.

I recall an experience with ayahuasca when unitive consciousness had transitioned into an awareness of a personal observer who was viewing a bird's-eye perspective of a medieval mountainside, filled with winding paths, forests, fields, streets, and houses and occupied by hundreds of people and animals, all busily going about their simple daily routines. What was so amazing in this particular state of consciousness was that I could choose to zero in and carefully observe individual people in the scene. I did this repeatedly, selecting different men, women, children, and even animals. I could see not only color and form, but detailed facial expressions and even the intricate designs on the fabric of women's dresses and lace accessories. It was like viewing a painting of a medieval scene in incredibly sharp focus that had become totally alive. If you ask how to understand such an experience, I haven't a clue. One could suggest that it was a memory from a prior lifetime, a God's-eye view of a particular scene in human history, or a manifestation of creative resources I never knew I possessed that conceivably someday could be expressed in a painting or by writing a novel. That it happened, however, remains vividly in my memory and contributes to the profound awe I experience concerning the potentials of human consciousness. I have known vivid or lucid dreams, some that were "dreams within dreams" in which one recognizes the dreaming process, that contained similar detail, but never with this degree of conscious control and focus, and never with such clear, enduring memory.

EMERGING WISDOM

The philosophical term "entelechy" refers to a purposive, meaningful process of unfolding content within awareness. In visionary states, quite in contrast to the fleeting visual phenomena typically encountered when psychedelics are ingested in relatively low dosage, the images and thematic progressions that lead one toward and into mystical consciousness and that appear as the ego subsequently begins to become reconstituted are often experienced not as random, but as creatively choreographed. Sometimes it is as though they illustrate personally potent story lines like those unfolding within a skillfully written novel. The very manner in which these experiential sequences present themselves is often described as exquisitely beautiful, their manifestation typically appearing to constitute evidence of a skillful and compassionate wisdom within our minds. This dynamic is often described as the divine coming to the individual human life and working effectively within it to effect personal teachings, redemption, or transformation. This is reflected in the respectful reference to ayahuasca and to peyote as "the Teacher." *Psilocybe cubensis*, a well-known species of sacred or magic mushrooms, is often called "The golden teacher."

So, to recapitulate and summarize here, let us note again that the intuitive knowledge often intrinsic to mystical forms of consciousness typically includes insights pertaining to (1) God, (2) Immortality, (3) Interrelatedness, (4) Love, (5) Beauty, and (6) Emerging Wisdom. In the mystical states that we consider "complete," "all the above" and more seem to apply.

FRUITS FOR LIFE

In thinking about whether mystical consciousness should be considered irrational or nonrational, it is also helpful to consider the "fruits for life" that often appear to follow its occurrence. Those who remember this profound dimension of human experience often report a feeling of progressive integration in the months and years afterward.

As time moves forward, they may claim to feel more compassionate, more tolerant of others, more creative, more courageous, and more self-accepting and at peace within themselves. Such claims now can be studied in research frameworks through follow-up interviews and psychological testing, both of the people who report mystical experiences and of the close friends and family members who observe their attitudes and behavior on a daily basis. Initial scientific confirmation of this phenomenon has been found in the Hopkins studies to date, notably Katherine MacLean's statistical discovery of positive changes in the domain of personality structure called Openness following mystical experiences. This is a striking development, since until recently most personality theorists have believed that the domains that structure our personalities are quite indelibly fixed by the time we arrive at adulthood. Undoubtedly, such positive effects can be nurtured and reinforced by spiritual disciplines and other life activities that one may choose to follow after the occurrence of the mystical experiences themselves.

An existential psychiatrist and philosopher, Karl Jaspers, coined the term "the unconditioned imperative" (*die unbedingte Forderung*) to refer to the experience of love, bubbling up like a spring, deep within the human mind. He understood it to be discovered and encountered in the experiential depths, often amid struggles with guilt and grief when glimpses of the sacred that he called "Transcendence" occurred. This could well be viewed as the love of God, called *agape* by theologians, that not only heals those who experience it, but also demands expression in and through their lives in interaction with other people and the world.

Similarly, St. Augustine of Hippo (354–430 CE), perhaps writing out of mystical experiences of his own, is reputed to have said, "Love and do as you will. If you keep silence, do it out of love. If you cry out, do it out of love." In modern language, one could acknowledge the sanctity of expression of both "tender love" and "tough love."

People who have known mystical consciousness, at least in their more centered states of mind, may be viewed by some as radiating a presence, wisdom, compassion, or power beyond themselves, manifested in diverse ways ranging from loving in gentle and intimate ways to risking one's life for a cause of social justice.

The image of the great Indian seer Ramana Maharshi may be illustrative. As described by the journalist Paul Brunton in his book *A Search in Secret India*, published in 1935, Ramana sits silently on his tiger skin, surrounded by disciples and visitors who claim to feel spiritually nurtured and healed, simply by being in his presence. As Ramana Maharshi may illustrate the "Being" pole of a compassionate continuum, so perhaps Mother Teresa may illustrate the "Doing" pole in her social activism in the slums of Calcutta. If indeed love of this magnitude dwells in the depths of each of us, a basis for ethics may be understood to be hardwired, perhaps genetically encoded, within the human organism. Healing in depth psychotherapy may be correspondingly viewed as approaching and dissolving the obstacles within to strengthen the connection with this inner source of love.

INCREASING TOLERANCE AND UNDERSTANDING

Perhaps we all inevitably grow up with stereotypes, regardless of our culture of origin. I recall an experience in the beautiful heights of northern India with fragrant pine forests and crystal-clear, cascading streams. There I visited an abandoned Anglican church, built of stone in Gothic architecture, left behind by the British when India became an independent nation. The old church was located in McLeodganj, now a predominantly Buddhist area near the Dalai Lama's compound where prayer flags flutter in the wind, and I walked in. It was in disrepair, no longer had a priest or congregation, and had become a tourist attraction. My visit happened to occur in spring, actually on Ash Wednesday, the first day of the Christian liturgical season of Lent. A Buddhist tour guide met me, invited a contribution, and proceeded to plug in a string of miniature colored lights on a dusty artificial Christmas tree to illustrate "what Christians do."

Similarly, having grown up in a somewhat conservative Christian atmosphere with the idea that members of Eastern religions tend to sit around gazing at their navels, quite insensitive to social needs and injustices, I was jolted into sanity when I visited the Sikh Golden Temple in the Indian city of Amritsar. Never have I witnessed such a well-organized, cooperative venture for providing free meals to people– literally feeding over forty thousand pilgrims and visitors every day of the year (and as many as one hundred thousand on holidays), coupled with impeccable cleanliness, almost constant music, and the sharing of their sacrament, or Prasad, with anyone who comes to worship, crossing the bridge over the sacred lake and entering the glistening temple. The good will and joy in the temple compound were contagious and I found myself sitting cross-legged on the ground with other volunteers around the edge of a large white sheet, busily helping to make chapattis.

In India, people greet one another with "Namaste," meaning, "I honor the divine within you." My impression was that many people in India, regardless of their specific religious identities, genuinely feel this sense of interpersonal connection and relatedness. The shared spirituality, whether Hindu, Jain, Buddhist, Muslim, Sikh, Jewish, Christian, or Zoroastrian, was palpable. Commitment to any religious tradition and practice appeared to be acceptable and respected. Perhaps what might be pitied or merit disapproval would be total religious disengagement and a lack of commitment and identity.

5

Approaches to
Unitive Consciousness

We now shift our focus from the intuitive insights often reported by people who have experienced mystical states of consciousness to zero in on the claims of an ultimate unity or oneness in the core, or at the ultimate source of Being. For the moment, let us set aside unique theological formulations, whether Eastern or Western. As noted previously "Atman is Brahman" and "Hear, O Israel, the Lord Thy God is One" could well be viewed as verbalizations in the wake of the same ultimate form of awareness, though the reverberating echoes of subsequent theological traditions and formulations in the East and the West have tended to be significantly divergent.

I recall serving on the thesis committee of a graduate student who was writing on the deepest levels of spiritual experience. Appreciating how ineffable the topic she had chosen was, I wondered if her final product would be a single piece of paper (high-quality embossed parchment, of course)–perhaps with the sacred symbol "Om" drawn calligraphically with India ink in the center. Somehow, as is expected for doctoral dissertations, however, she still managed to come up with several hundred pages of English words.

Although perhaps we are rendered speechless and wordless by unitive consciousness itself, it is possible to find some words to speak or write about two ways in which it seems to be approached. Studying the historical literature of works written by mystics of the past, the philosopher Walter Stace formulated two approaches to unity that he called Introvertive and Extrovertive. Walter Pahnke and I preferred to use the terms "Internal Unity" and "External Unity." Whether or not the ultimate unity approached in either way is the same is one of those issues some scholars enjoy debating; I for one am content to view unity as unity. A psychologist of religion, Ralph Hood, who developed a psychological test for documenting the occurrence of mystical experiences that he administered to both Christian and Jewish mystics in the United States and also to Islamic mystics in Iran, was able to find empirical support for these two different descriptions of unitive consciousness.

INTERNAL UNITY

Internal Unity is most commonly reported in the psilocybin research at the Johns Hopkins School of Medicine, as volunteers usually recline on a couch in a comfortable living-room type of setting and wear a sleep-shade and headphones during most of the time period when the entheogen is active. The sleep-shade is intended to block out environmental distractions while the headphones provide supportive music, usually selections carefully chosen from the classical repertoire. With closed eyes, one typically reports a sense of subjective movement through various so-called dimensions of being, while awareness of one's everyday personality fades even though consciousness continues, until a mystical experience occurs, or as some might poetically say, until mystical consciousness announces and affirms itself. This movement tends to be more passive than active, as if one is being summoned or drawn toward mystical illumination. One chooses to entrust oneself to more fundamental levels of being, often an act of unconditional trust and surrender by a healthy ego. The old stereotype depicted by some theologians of a heroic ego, inflated with its self-importance, trying to charge through the gates of heaven with upraised sword to claim the holy grail of enlightenment is clearly simply "an old stereotype." In truth, the everyday self or ego, humbly and unconditionally, must choose to trust, receive, and participate with all that is emerging from within the depths of the mind.

This threshold between the personal (that is, the everyday self) and the transpersonal (that is, more fundamental or universal dimensions of consciousness) is conceptualized by different people in different ways. Most commonly, the term "death" is employed as the ego (everyday self) feels that it quite literally is dying. Though one may have read that others have reported subsequent immersion in the eternal and experiences of being reborn and returning to everyday existence afterward, in the moment imminence of death may feel acutely–and for some terrifyingly–real. The challenge is to trust unconditionally and to simply allow death to occur. This requires faith, not solely as the rational acceptance of the tenets of a religious creed, but as a courageous act of trust. The Danish theologian Søren Kierkegaard expressed this experiential act as "the leap of faith." It is somewhat akin to diving headfirst off of a high diving board, trusting that there is indeed water of sufficient depth in the pool below. Clearly, this act for many can occur more easily when one is in a medical or religious setting with trusted companions and when the purity and dosage of the entheogen are known.

An alternative to conceptualizing this transition as death is, amid relinquishing control, feeling that one is "going crazy" and then choosing with the supportive presence of one's guide to let it happen and "go crazy." This transition in consciousness, even with momentary panic and sometimes fear and suspiciousness, can rapidly give way to a sense of being "at home" deep within one's mind. It commonly is reported not that the experiential world becomes increasingly weird and surreal as one relinquishes the controls of the ego and goes deeper, but the converse–that one feels increasingly centered and at peace. Some people call it "homecoming," feel welcomed by parts of their minds they hardly knew existed, and report a familiar sense of "having been there before." A common verbal expression is, "Of course, it always has been this way," often accompanied by feelings of joy and even laughter at the thought that one ever could have doubted or forgotten this fundamental sense of belonging in the universe.

Still others may describe the ascent (or descent if you prefer) to mystical realms of consciousness as "melting" or "dissolving," even as being deliciously seduced by a divine lover. Occasionally someone may feel that energies are building up stronger, stronger, and even stronger and that one is about to explode into countless fragments. Just as the supportive counsel would be to accept what one has labeled death, going crazy, melting, or dissolving, so here it would be to allow the "explosion" to occur. The bottom line with a well-prepared person is to trust one's own mind, one's grounding with the guide beside him or her, the safety of the physical surroundings, and, if religious perspectives permit, God or another sacred symbol for ultimate reality. In this context, there really is nothing to fear. The mind may undergo one or more intense experiences of death and rebirth and awareness of the ego (that is, that part of your mind that functions with your name in everyday life) may ebb and flow. Similarly, awareness of the body lying on the couch may come and go as one might expect to experience in a state of deep trance. However, the heart and lungs will continue to function steadily.

A metaphor that some have found useful in conceptualizing this approach to unity is found in a spherical amoeba–that single-celled microorganism that most of us peered at through microscopes in our high school biology classes. The spherical cell may well symbolize the unitive nature of mystical consciousness. However, amoebas also develop pseudopods, strings of cytoplasm that are like "false feet" that gradually extend outward from the cell. Like the ego venturing into time and then retreating from time in cycles of birth and growth followed by old age and death, the pseudopod exists for a while, and then is drawn back into the spherical cell, vanishes, and is no longer part of the organism itself. A similar metaphor is the Hindu concept of the ego as a drop of water that ceases to exist as a separate being when it falls into the ocean and becomes an integral part of something much larger than itself. If the word "existence" pertains to awareness in time and "essence" is understood to describe the eternal dimensions of consciousness, then it makes sense for one to say, "I ceased to exist, but recall a state of mind of pure 'is-ness,' essence, or primal being."

In illustration, here is one description by a middle-aged woman with a history of kidney cancer from the report of her psilocybin session:

Early on the visuals came and dissolved so quickly I could not verbalize them in time . . . there were countless variations in what reminded me of the ceiling of Westminster Abby: gothic, vaulted, with great intricacy. These images changed lighting, color, and texture. . . . I had no doubt I was in the presence of the Infinite because I felt an overriding peacefulness that carried me through everything, even the very few seconds of "Yikes!" that showed up. I had a sense of losing my observer. I no longer witnessed the images. I was becoming them. This was not exactly creepy, but I did hesitate a minute, feeling my way slowly. There was a sense of being engulfed. "Am I about to be possessed, is this okay?" I love this bit: I was unwilling to just hand over my body. I said, "If we do this I want my body returned to me in at least as good a shape as it is in now." The reply came, "Do you think I would disrespect my own handiwork?" I got the point and went with it. . . . My body lit up, all parts in succession. It was the brightest thing I have ever seen. I glowed brilliantly from within. My whole being fluttered. I felt I was being breathed through or played like an instrument. Stunningly beautiful. I got that every part of all of us is sacred. There is no speck in the cosmos which is apart from this breath. The point of it all is sheer pleasure. The world is a misery out of love, presenting us with constant opportunities to find our way home. . . . I am seeing myself in everybody, and everybody in myself.

This woman's shift in inner perspective–expressed in "Do you think I would disrespect my own handiwork?"–resonates well with the well-known poem "Love" written by the British writer George Herbert in the early seventeenth century, which begins as follows:

LOVE bade me welcome; yet my soul drew back,
Guilty of dust and sin.
But quick-eyed Love, observing me grow slack
From my first entrance in,
Drew nearer to me, sweetly questioning
If I lack'd anything.

"A guest," I answer'd, "worthy to be here":
Love said, "You shall be he."
"I, the unkind, ungrateful? Ah, my dear,

I cannot look on Thee."
Love took my hand and smiling did reply,
"Who made the eyes but I?"

Another illustration is from the psilocybin report of a man with lung cancer whose religious orientation was Tibetan Buddhist:

There were several visual transformations and I was amazed at how subtle and gradual the transformations were–not abrupt, fast, or disorienting but very comfortable and gentle–changing almost imperceptibly slowly. . . . Gradually my experience of a higher plane of consciousness deepened and was associated with a gradual change of my vision from a fabric connecting all of our consciousnesses to all of our consciousnesses being together as a unified consciousness in a warm, enclosed space, almost like a womb. I had the deepening awareness that I had fully experienced a sort of enlightened state in which I was clearly aware of the interrelationship of all phenomena and sentient beings and that I was in a consciousness that transcended the ordinary state that I could remember from the session room when we started. . . . Next began a period of deepening awe at the depth of my experience of enlightenment, a feeling of natural omniscience without any hint of ego or pride . . . I had transformation after transformation of my consciousness that appeared to present me with a complete understanding of myriads of situations and phenomena, why individuals have afflictive emotions, why I felt emotionally connected to all other sentient beings, how world leaders come to power, sickness, old age, death, past, present, future. I cannot articulate *what* my understanding of these was at that time, only that I was convinced that I had a complete understanding of all these and countless other subjects–a feeling of benevolent omniscience . . .

Though I do not believe in a creator "God" outside of us which is self- existent, or existent independent of our own cognition, I feel this session brought me to the God experience, whatever that means. I do not feel "I became one with God," or "I reached out and touched God," but rather that I had the deep feeling of *becoming* God for what was actually a short time but seemed like millennia.

A third illustration is from the LSD experience of a man suffering from alcoholism:

> The most emotional experience I had during the day was the feeling as though I had died and was drifting into space–moving away from the earth. I started to become very uneasy and nervous and then the clouds seemed to move aside for me to pass. I was terribly frightened. I felt so alone out there all by myself. Sometimes I seemed to be moving much faster–the clouds parting more swiftly. I wanted very much to go back but knew I could not. I began to drift more slowly now and had become more calm. The clouds had gone by.
>
> From here on it is very difficult to explain. There was nothing. It was like slowly drifting into empty space. It was so beautifully bright you could see nothing. Then far off a small cloud or a flower appeared. The beauty and colors were so intense. It brought tears to my eyes, but I could not turn away from it. I stretched out my arms to encircle it, but it was growing like a beautiful flower. It became larger and larger until I could no longer control it. Then it seemed to burst into such magnificence and beauty as everything seemed to open up. I was laughing at the happiness it gave me. I screamed as I pointed. (It's so beautiful you can't see it.) At that time I thought I was God, but I couldn't be. This was God and this must be heaven. I became very confused again. If God were here and I was here . . .
>
> I was God. God was me at that time–it seemed all men were here. We must truly all be one. I thought this is what has been said of eternal life.

The limitations of language become especially constricting when one attempts to express unitive states of consciousness. There may well be many degrees of intensity or completeness encountered by different people, or by the same person at different times. For example, one person may write of experiencing himself or herself as one atom in the lotus throne that supports the Buddha and being profoundly grateful to "simply be a part" of something so profoundly sacred. Another may describe humbly being one of thousands of bodhisattvas surrounding the Buddha. Yet another may speak–or hesitate to speak–of entering into the eternal essence of Buddhahood. Similar varieties of expression are reported in a framework of Christian traditions and imagery. What is common in all these experiences is a sense of the merging of the everyday personality, often called the ego, with spiritual reality that intuitively feels more fundamental and all encompassing.

EXTERNAL UNITY

In meditative disciplines, there is a tradition of letting one's gaze rest on a single point, simply "being with" the perception. Though the object on which one chooses to focus could be most anything, common choices are a candle flame, the center of a mandala, or an individual flower. With or without the aid of entheogens, the flower, for example, sometimes may appear to change in form or hue over time, often seeming to open as in time-lapse photography. There may be a series of intriguing perceptual changes for a while and then, in rare instances, a shift of perception is reported, accompanied by a noetic insight that "all is one." Here is a description from the personal report of an LSD-assisted experience:

> There were profound feelings of unity, first with a red tulip, and then with a rose of the same color. When looking at the rose as an object, it seemed to come alive before my eyes. Its petals seemed to breathe as, slowly and gracefully, they unfolded, seeming to express the ultimate in beauty. Fascinated, I watched these movements of cosmic gentleness until, suddenly, I *knew* the rose; that is to say, I somehow became One with the rose, no longer existing as an ego passively viewing an object in its environment. Although in the objectivity of my critical mind I knew there were no physical changes in the flower, subjectively I seemed to see it in a totally new perspective, one which elicited tears and deep feelings of reverence. The rose seemed to stand out in naked beauty, as though it were the only thing existing in the world.

Supporting the ancient monistic school of thought, I expressed the philosophical insight that "we are all the same thing." Once I sought to express my experience by speaking of "becoming one with the very essence of Roseness." Another time I commented that, "There is more to beauty than we know."

And here is one more illustration, this one by Aldous Huxley in *The Doors of Perception* as he tried to describe unity triggered by focusing on the leg of a bamboo table:

I was looking at my furniture, not as the utilitarian who has to sit on chairs, to write at desks and tables, and not as the camera-man or scientific recorder, but as the pure aesthete whose concern is only with forms and their relationships within the field of vision or the picture space. But as I looked this purely aesthetic, Cubist's-eye view gave place to what I can only describe as the sacramental vision of reality. I was back where I had been when I was looking at the flowers–back in a world where everything shone with the Inner Light, and was infinite in its significance. The legs, for example, of that chair–how miraculous their tubularity, how supernatural their polished smoothness! I spent several minutes–or was it several centuries?–not merely gazing at those bamboo legs, but actually *being* them–or rather being myself in them; or, to be still more accurate (for "I" was not involved in the case, nor in a certain sense were "they") being my Not-self in the Not-self which was the chair.

Though both of these illustrations focus on the sense of vision with eyes wide open, it appears that unity may also be approached through other sensory modalities, sometimes with reports of having become one with music. Here is one description from a psilocybin session of how music may be experienced as enhanced perception approaches mystical awareness:

The various pieces of music were wonderful, because they were multi-dimensional. I could hear tiny variations and subtle changes and shadings in the voices and instruments, as if I were inside the mind of the composer as HE heard it. There was the sense of the composer touching the divine and channeling its perfection down to the human level, so that other people could be aware of it and uplifted, too, but simultaneous awareness of the impossibility of the task, as imperfect human beings, imperfect instruments, and imperfect voices are involved. Somehow all of that imperfection was also woven into the perfection the music was channeling. I was inside the music, the composer, the players, the singers, the shaft of the woodwind, the metal keys of the woodwinds, and the finger pressing the keys.

Another volunteer expressed her experience of the relationship of her everyday personality and mystical union in a metaphor of a cosmic symphony orchestra with countless musicians in which she experienced herself as one of thousands in the third clarinet section. As an individual player, or ego, she could contribute an infinitesimal part to the magnificence of the music if she played her best, but it was abundantly clear that, no matter how she played, she did not have the power to detract from the beauty of the symphony as a whole. It was; she was part of it; and in the unitive awareness all she was and all she ever could do were encompassed in music of infinite dimensions. A similar metaphor is the ego as one grain of sand and mystical consciousness as all the deserts, dunes, beaches, and ocean floors of the world.

Poetic as it may sound, the best description of the approach and occurrence of external unity I have heard depicts the perceiver and the perceived meeting on an atomic or subatomic level of experiencing, in which the atoms and subatomic "particles" that make up the perceiver and the atoms and subatomic "particles" that make up the object of perception somehow resonate with one another, triggering an awareness that ultimately the world that we perceive and we ourselves are made up of the same "stuff" in one great unity. The British mathematician and philosopher Alfred North Whitehead may be understood to have been trying to express something of this nature when he wrote of "prehension," which he defined as "uncognitive apprehension." The most common word choice to express this profoundly insightful experience appears to be the simple phrase "all is one."

Experiences of external unity may well occur more frequently when one's body is outside in a natural setting, especially when one's eyes are open. When high dosage and ego transcendence are involved, walking in the world entails some risk and it would be especially important to have a trusted guide beside one to ensure physical safety. Research with entheogens tends to be conducted in interior spaces, where one's body can safely sink into a couch and the mind can be freed from having to "watch over the body."

In the early period of psychedelic research in Maryland, conducted at the Maryland Psychiatric Research Center, located on the spacious campus of the Spring Grove Hospital Center, the first hours of sessions would be conducted on a couch in an interior treatment suite, but, weather permitting, in the final hours guides would take volunteers for walks outside. Many persons would lean against an ancient old tree on the campus and, in varying degrees, identify with its strength or claim to become it. Entering into it in symbolically meaningful ways, some would report feeling their legs penetrating like roots deep into the earth and their arms rising and stretching heavenward like branches.

6

New Perspectives
on Time and Space

This chapter is written to highlight the category called Transcendence of Time and Space included in the definition of mystical consciousness. I am not trained in theoretical physics and barely begin to adequately comprehend the philosophy of Immanuel Kant, who pondered the mysteries of time and space long and hard back in the eighteenth century. Others, more qualified than I, have written and will write their own books about the mysteries of matter and how its deepest substrates appear to behave differently than our sensory perceptions and usual styles of thinking would lead us to expect or even conceive as within the realm of possibility.

Huston Smith eloquently expressed this mind-boggling dilemma of our intellects in the essay "The Revolution in Western Thought," published in 1961 in the *Saturday Evening Post* and reprinted in his book *Beyond the Post-Modern Mind*:

> If modern physics showed us a world at odds with our senses, postmodern physics is showing us one which is at odds with our imagination. . . . That the table which appears motionless

is in fact incredibly "alive" with electrons circling their nuclei a million billion times per second; that the chair which feels so secure beneath us is actually a near vacuum–such facts, while certainly very strange, posed no permanent problem for man's sense of order. To accommodate them, all that was necessary was to replace the earlier picture of a gross and ponderous world with a subtle world in which all was sprightly dance and airy whirl.

But the problems the new physics poses for man's sense of order cannot be resolved by refinements in scale. Instead they appear to point to a radical disjunction between the way things behave and every possible way in which we might try to visualize them. How, for example, are we to picture an electron traveling two or more different routes through space concurrently, or passing from orbit to orbit without traversing the intervening space? What kind of model can we construct of a space that is finite yet unbounded, or of light which is both wave and particle? It is such enigmas which have caused physicists like P. W. Bridgman of Harvard to suggest that "the structure of nature may eventually be such that our processes of thought do not correspond to it sufficiently to permit us to think about it at all. . . . The world fades out and eludes us. . . . We are confronted with something truly ineffable. We have reached the limit of the vision of the great pioneers of science, the vision, namely, that we live in a sympathetic world in that it is comprehensible by our minds."

We all can understand that time and space clearly contribute to the organization of our lives in normal waking consciousness. Temporal experiences are catalogued in three files: past, present, and future–the third, we usually assume, includes potential, planned, unexpected, and unknowable experiences. At birth, we "discover ourselves in the world" (in the words of the existentialist Martin Heidegger), then live out our lives year by year as we age, experiencing many of the joys and pains of human existence, and finally arrive at death, that point of either cessation or transition of consciousness that comes to us all. We move through space from home to work, walking, driving, or flying from one city to another, or even through outer space to the moon or other planets. There are fairly reliable mathematics involved in all this as our trusty GPS demonstrates.

What is so perplexing is that people who have mystical experiences often claim not only that they were distracted or unaware of the passing of time, but that the state of consciousness they were experiencing was intuitively felt to be "outside of time." In many alternate states of consciousness, with and without the assistance of entheogens, time may be experienced as slowed down or speeded up. If asked how much clock time has elapsed during a psychedelic session, one sometimes may make a very inaccurate estimate, in one direction or the other. We all experience this to some extent when we experience time passing rapidly when we are immersed in activities we enjoy and, conversely, we all know how slowly time can pass when we're bored. For this writer, gardening, hiking in nature, or performing music usually entails decreased awareness of time; conversely, when I am waiting in long lines or stalled in heavy traffic seconds can feel like minutes. In his studies of highly self-actualizing people, Abraham Maslow called attention to reports of altered time perception amid creative fervor, when a poet or artist becomes "oblivious of his surroundings and the passage of time." Perhaps these changes in time perception may be understood as precursory transitions to the mystical transcendence of time in which consciousness awakens to eternal dimensions, akin to a plane taking off on a rainy day, gradually penetrating through thick layers of clouds and then finally breaking through into a realm of dazzling blue sky and sunlight.

Space is similarly claimed to be transcended in mystical states. The heavenly realms are not experienced as located in a particular place, either in our universe or in another galaxy, like some vacation spot where one could send a spaceship if we knew the vectors to program in a targeted address. Rather, mystical consciousness is claimed to be "everywhere and nowhere" and space simply seems to be a concept that works well as we think and function in the everyday world of sense perception, but that somehow is either incorporated or left behind in the eternal realms.

This is true not only of visionary experiences, but of the contents of our fields of awareness in everyday existence. Is there a location for the thought you are having right now, the dream you recall from last night, or a memory from your childhood? Might it be found hiding microscopically encoded in a corner of one of the billions of cells in your nervous system? Searching for such a location might be as futile and inappropriate as examining a transistor from a television set in search of the attractive blonde woman who appeared on the screen last night and delivered the weather report during the evening news. In the final analysis, now in the early twenty-first century, we honestly do not know what we are, and it is very hard to think without reference to time, space, and substance. However, when all is said and done, even when we stare, with or without powerful microscopes, perplexed at the grey matter and white matter that comprise our central nervous systems, striving to comprehend our physiology as best we can, we do know *that* we are and that there are experiential contents within our minds.

Dare we take seriously claims that, from the perspective of the Eternal Now, it might actually be possible to travel into the past, to recall not only the details of childhood events, but even prior lifetimes? Is it really conceivable that we may be capable of reliving fetal development or the evolution of our species as some have claimed? Books by Jean Houston and Robert Masters and by Stanislav Grof describe very unique experiences that stretch our imaginations regarding what might be possible, even extending into communication with nonhuman life forms. Those who have transcended space in mystical states have not uncommonly suggested that the universes we probe in astronomy and those we probe in microbiology ultimately somehow might be one and the same.

In terms of time perception, consider whether it might actually be possible to glimpse where the saga of history is heading and have valid, precognitive insights either of what may be determined or of what potentially may happen if we don't affirm our freedom and act to change things. When a person claims to "remember the future," should we quickly refer him or her for psychiatric care or respectfully honor the potential validity of experiential knowledge we still have no way of comprehending? Parapsychologists have been documenting examples of precognition for a long time, but their findings are so difficult to comprehend in the context of our dominant view of the nature of reality that they are still rarely given serious attention.

WALTER PAHNKE'S INITIATION
AND POSSIBLE PREMONITION

Returning to the life of my friend Walter Pahnke, introduced in chapter 3, let me add that, to the surprise of no one who knew him, once the award of his PhD was finally confirmed by Harvard University, he allowed himself to personally explore the effects of a psychedelic substance. The first occasion was an LSD session in Hanscarl Leuner's clinic in Göttingen, Germany, on February 29, 1964. I found myself being a supportive presence with him, returning the favor he had done for me only two weeks earlier. In my journal that evening, I wrote: "His ecstatic shouts still ring in my ears: 'Beauty, Oh!, I can't believe it! Fantastic! Oh! I never could have imagined. Wow! Fantaaastic! Man, this is great! I never would have thought. . . . Joy, blessing, tenderness. Oh, Bill–this is great! You can't imagine–Oh yes you can.'"

In subsequent years, we sometimes spoke of two styles of ecstasy, one extrovertive and explosive, one introvertive and quiet. Wally's first experience clearly illustrated the former. Later in that same journal entry, I continued: "Near the end we spoke of many things, not least the sense of personal destiny we both feel to some degree. I have a feeling Wally and I may really work together someday. The same destiny that brought us together this time may well bring us together in the future, guiding two pioneers in a fantastic expedition. We feel such awe, such wonder, such humility in the midst of our joy." Actually, we were able to collaborate in some research with psilocybin in Boston, along with the anthropologist Richard Katz and the psychiatrist Carl Salzman, in 1966, two years later–also the year I married with Wally standing beside me as my best man. Then we both moved to Baltimore in 1967 where we worked together in psychedelic research at the Spring Grove Hospital Center and then at the Maryland Psychiatric Research Center, especially devoted to exploring how entheogens in the context of brief psychotherapy might help terminal cancer patients to live more fully.

Then, after four years of collaborative psychedelic research in Baltimore, along with other intrepid investigators including Albert Kurland, Charles Savage, Sanford Unger, Stanislav Grof, Robert Soskin, Sidney Wolf, Lee McCabe, and others, I received a late-evening phone call on July 10, 1971. Sadly, I was informed that Wally had gone scuba diving, alone in the rocky ocean waters in front of his cabin near Bath, Maine, and had not resurfaced. Stunned, I hung up the phone and said to my wife, "Wally is dead." The Coast Guard continued to trawl for his body during the night and into the next day. It never has been recovered.

In light of his death, the report he wrote of that first LSD experience of his in Germany fuels some of the awe and curiosity I experience when I ponder the mystery of time. His verbatim words with his own capitalization and underlining were as follows:

> The most impressive and intense part of this experience was the WHITE LIGHT of absolute purity and cleanness. It was like a glowing and sparkling flame of incandescent whiteness and beauty, but not really a flame–more like a gleaming white hot ingot, yet much bigger and vaster than a mere ingot. The associated feelings were those of *absolute* AWE, REVERENCE, AND SACREDNESS. Just before this experience I had the feeling of going deep within myself to the Self stripped bare of all pretense and falseness. This was the point where a man could stand firm with absolute integrity–something more important than mere physical life. The white light experience was of *supreme importance*–absolutely self validating and something worth staking your life on and putting your trust in. The white light itself was so penetrating and intense that it was not possible to look directly at it. It was not in the room with me, but we were both somewhere else–and my body was left far behind.
>
> Later, I again went deep within myself, and I had the image of going down deep into a dark, silent pool. Then I had a vision of absolute DIVINE love. It was like a flowing spring of silvery white liquid overflowing upward and was very beautiful to watch and feel. The feeling was of love and compassion toward the Divine and toward all men. I had the insight that all men had this same potential and worth within themselves. All men were equal in the sight of God and to my own feelings at this moment. I realized how I had not taken this enough into account in my past actions.

I knew Wally to be an exceptionally brilliant man who did indeed manifest absolute integrity. He seemed to want to optimize every moment of every day, as if he somehow always knew that his life-span was limited. I recall repeatedly running behind him down several flights of stairs, two steps at a time, to arrive at the cafeteria of the Massachusetts Mental Health Center seconds before it closed, and finally choosing to accept and affirm my own pace in life, which was considerably slower. In a foreign city, he'd want to visit all the tourist attractions in one afternoon; I'd tend to be content with exploring one or two wings of a single museum. He'd drive miles out of his way to find gasoline a few pennies cheaper or to obtain a free colorful drinking glass filled with cottage cheese. He always insisted on cutting his own hair in a mirror—sometimes with rather questionable outcomes!

In spite of his medical training and academic brilliance, Wally was also accident-prone. I remember him coming to work on crutches and hobbling down hallways during at least two different periods of time. He knew he suffered from what might be called a "spoiled only child syndrome" and that sometimes he could be quite preoccupied with his own agendas and insensitive to the needs of family, friends, and colleagues. Finally, refusing to wait a few minutes longer to be joined by his wife, he put on scuba gear he had borrowed from a friend (never having gone scuba diving before), dove into the Atlantic Ocean, and vanished, leaving behind his wife, parents, and three children between the ages of two and ten. Was he brilliant or stupid?

Wally was certainly considered smart, as evidenced by his many degrees, his many accomplishments, and his 99th percentile scores on the Graduate Record Examination. Yet emotionally he was crippled and was desperately trying to slow down and bond more with his family. My wife lovingly called him "an intellectual giant and an emotional dwarf." When I spoke at his memorial service in Baltimore, I acknowledged that everyone who loved Wally had also been angry with him and I observed many heads nodding in expressions of agreement. While some have speculated about suicidal intent, I knew him well enough to accept his death as evidence of mere impulsiveness and the reckless stupidity of an otherwise brilliant man.

But here is the crux—the enigma that my mind sometimes ponders in the middle of the night: No other volunteer in my experience has ever described "a flowing spring of silvery white liquid overflowing upward" during a psychedelic session, though "going down deep into a dark, silent pool" may be somewhat more consonant with the usual repertoire of images of sacred experiences. Together, the two phrases are certainly suggestive of bubbles from a tank of compressed air at the time of his death and the descent of his body into a dark crevice in the ocean's depths, though that simply could be a strange coincidence. Right . . . or?

Wally's LSD experience with its possibly precognitive sequence occurred in 1964 at age thirty-three; his death occurred in 1971 at age forty. I have wondered if it was his destiny, determined to occur no matter what he did in terms of personal growth, and if he somehow had a glimpse of the future in his LSD session. Or was a potential end of his life revealed to him along with the freedom to alter the trajectory he was on? If the latter is the case, perhaps he failed to emotionally mature fast enough and finally took one chance too many. Maybe some disciplinary principle in the universe ruled: "That's it! No more chances." Or perhaps he was simply born with a forty-year lifespan, uniquely perfect in its design. He did make his contributions to the world.

To add to the mystery, thirty-six days before his death, Wally arrived at work seriously shaken by a dream from the night before in which he had jumped out of a plane without a parachute. As a man who rarely remembered dreams, its intensity and dominance in his field of consciousness surprised and concerned him. He wrote the dream down and gave me a copy: "As I fell nearer to what I thought was the end of my life, I felt an overpowering feeling of disgust at my misjudgment or stupidity–I need not have jumped without a parachute–what was I thinking of–how did I ever think I could have gotten away with it? . . . As I drove to work I kept thinking about the dream–couldn't get it out of my mind. It seemed very vivid–more so than almost any dream I can remember."

As in a child's "choose your own adventure" book, Wally reported that his dream had four different endings:

I for a short time had split level consciousness–I hit the ground with a terrific impact and then I was falling again. I seemed to live through different outcomes: (1) the end with blackness; (2) the end, then spirit consciousness and presence at my funeral; (3) impact with splintered legs and prolonged hospitalization– an invalid or cripple; (4) impact–miraculous survival. I somehow escaped injury and walked away. One of those miracle landings that I have read about.

As these different possible endings alternated with falling it seemed that somehow the 4th ending had happened. What luck, yet almost too good to be true. Yet I was not too sure it had really happened–or had I just ended the dream before really finding out. This was unclear, but the latter seemed the case.

Philosophers have long pondered deterministic forces in life and how they may be balanced with human freedom. From the perspective of mystical consciousness, this may simply be one more of those paradoxes of "Both/And," where there is truth to be found in both perspectives and ultimate understanding continues to elude us. The best I have ever been able to verbalize when pondering this paradox is to conclude that perhaps we are determined to believe in the illusion of freedom, for if we do not act as though we are free, what is determined will fail to occur. Meanwhile, we live our lives and act in the world as best we can.

7

Visions and Archetypes

DEFINITIONS

In scholarly discussions in the psychology of religion, visions or vision-ary experiences tend to be distinguished from experiences of mystical consciousness, even though they often may seem to occur simultane-ously or one may flow into the other. This may seem to be a pedantic attempt to separate two incredibly profound and meaningful types of human experiences, but the distinction can enhance clarity of thought on this terrain at the frontiers of language. To recapitulate, mystical consciousness by definition includes unitive consciousness, preceded by the "death" of the individual personality and followed by its "rebirth," often accompanied by significant intuitive knowledge. In it the "subject -object dichotomy," a fancy philosophical term for the experience of feeling separate from what one is perceiving, is transcended or over-come. Visionary experiences, with either open or closed eyes, typically occur with the subject-object framework still intact: I am *here*, looking–even awesomely beholding–something *there*. I may see it, approach it, tremble before it, and relate to it with love or fear, but I do not fully "enter into it" or "become one with it." Such visionary experiences are often reported just prior to or just after experiences of unitive-mystical consciousness, but there are many instances when they stand on their own as the culmination of a particular journey into alternative realms of awareness. If visionary experiences are the apexes of foothills surrounding the mountainous peak of mystical consciousness that penetrates through, above, and beyond the clouds, they are still very impressive in themselves.

What one sees in visionary experiences are often called "archetypes." This term can be traced back to Philo of Alexandria, a Greek philosopher who lived from 20 BCE to 40 CE. The term was reclaimed by the Swiss psychiatrist Carl Gustav Jung (1875–1961), who, on the basis of his own dream imagery and that of his patients, including both nocturnal memories and images actively evoked while lying on the analytic couch, posited a "collective unconscious" within each of our minds where archetypes may be encountered. They may simply be described as "foundation stones of our psychic structure" or as "the innate furnishings of our unconscious minds"–universal images that most, if not all of us, seem to share. Perhaps we are born with them, somehow encoded in our genes; perhaps we are able in special states of awareness to access them spiritually (whatever that may mean scientifically). "Stones" or "furnishings" are rather limiting terms to describe archetypes, however, as many of these images radiate incredible portentousness and power. They may be encountered with awe and perceived as intrinsically magnificent and meaningful. They influence, move, and inspire us. They may even seem to propel large social movements and the development of civilizations on the world stage.

Archetypes include gods and goddesses, precious gemstones and metals, angels and demons, and similar visionary content, not only recorded in the scriptures of our world's religions, but also encountered in alternative states of consciousness by men and women, still today with and without the use of entheogens. What is so fascinating in psychedelic research is the discovery that volunteers not uncommonly report visions of religious and cultural content that is unexpected and sometimes is claimed to be totally foreign to what they have learned in life thus far. John Locke, a seventeenth-century British philosopher, suggested that we come into the world with minds that are tabula rasa, "sheets of paper white on which anyone may write," akin to brand new computers waiting to be programmed. The findings from psychedelic research suggest that Locke was dead wrong and that he significantly underestimated the resources and mysteries within us. There are now sufficient data in the descriptive records of psychedelic researchers to consider Jung's concept of the collective unconscious empirically validated.

HINDU GODS IN A WESTERN MIND

I recall a research volunteer in his early twenties who had grown up in a poverty-stricken area of the inner city of Baltimore, who dropped out of junior high school, became addicted to heroin, and had been incarcerated in the Maryland prison system. He was paroled to live in a halfway house we operated for a research project exploring the promise of LSD in the treatment of narcotic addiction at that time, and I was able to give him a relatively high dose of LSD in the context of brief, intensive psychotherapy. When he dictated a report of his psychedelic experience, he described "strange, partially naked figures dancing with funny hats like crowns on their heads." A few days later, when he chanced upon a book of Hindu art in our waiting room before a follow-up appointment, he burst into my office, pointing excitedly at pictures of Vishnu and the dancing Shiva, saying with pressured speech, "This is what I saw; this is what I saw!" I remember pondering his experience that day, thinking how incredible it was, and how almost mundane it had become for those of us who were pursuing psychedelic research on a daily basis.

How did the dancing Shiva get into the mind of a culturally deprived, American narcotic addict? Of course, one can posit that he might have chanced upon the image while sitting in a barbershop as a child, perhaps leafing through an old *Life* or *Look* magazine, or perhaps he might have glimpsed it in one of the many television programs he had watched in his isolated childhood. But even that would not explain why, among all the images he may have seen in life, Hindu gods would make their appearance in his field of consciousness during an LSD session.

UNEXPECTED ENCOUNTERS

Similarly, the memory of an Australian psychiatrist comes to mind. This man had applied to participate in a program at the Maryland

Psychiatric Research Center that provided a legal experience with LSD for interested mental health and religious professionals. We called it our "Training Project." He hoped for some insight into what he called his "aboriginal roots" and claimed to have been "essentially uncontaminated" (his term) by Christianity.

His experience with LSD proved to be one of the most classically Christian dramas I have ever witnessed. After three days of stunned silence, he "confessed" not only that he had beheld the Christ, but that he had identified with him, experienced crucifixion and resurrection, and felt immersed in the love and unity of mystical consciousness. Were it not for his commitment to scholarship and intellectual honesty, his embarrassment about the nature of his experience might well have manifested in denial and a censored, incomplete report. One may theorize about how his original dislike and disregard of the little he knew about Christianity may have triggered a reaction formation, but regardless of his particular psychodynamic processes, this vignette stands out as a prime illustration of how people can experience content they find totally surprising during the action of entheogens.

The memory of the DPT session of another young narcotic addict from an impoverished neighborhood within the inner city of Baltimore comes to mind. Lying on his back on our white couch, securely nestled beneath blue flannel sheets, wearing an eyeshade and headphones as the entheogen was taking effect, he sensed he was rising into the heavens to meet God. He rose higher and higher and, as the clouds parted, suddenly he uttered a loud curse, tore off his eyeshade and headphones, threw off the sheets, sat up, looked me straight in the eye, and exclaimed, in alarm and dismay, "God's a woman!" His Baptist Sunday school clearly had not prepared him to cope with the divine in its feminine manifestation, either as the Great Mother, as the Virgin Mary, as Quan Yin (the Buddhist goddess of compassion), or as Fatima Zahra, in Islam. Yet the creative forces in his own mind apparently chose to introduce him to God in this manner.

TEONANÁCATYL

Another example of visionary experience comes from my own first experience with LSD, still in the clinic of Hanscarl Leuner in 1964. I had been volunteering in his clinic as a research assistant, preparing and supporting visiting English-speaking professionals who requested an opportunity to experience the effects of a major entheogen while the substances were still legal in Germany. In appreciation, Dr. Leuner was willing to allow me to investigate a few psychedelic substances beyond the scope of the original research project in which I had participated, trusting I would do so responsibly and write up good research reports afterward. After all, I was a graduate student in good physical and mental health, and the entheogens were understood to be essentially nontoxic and nonaddictive. In those days, believe it or not, there was no social stigma or controversy associated with psychedelics.

During this LSD session, when I took a break from lying prone with eyeshade and headphones, I sat on the edge of a couch with open eyes and chose to focus my attention on a replica of a Mazatec mushroom stone from the Rietberg Museum in Zurich that stood on the coffee table in front of me. This water-worn sculpture, as I recall it, was of an open, mature mushroom, originally carved out of sand-colored stone, perhaps one foot in height, with the face and body of a stylized ancient god with a headdress slightly emerging from the stalk or stem. As I concentrated on the sculpture, I found to my amazement, amusement, and delight that the god began to come alive before my eyes. His facial expression changed—sometimes serious, sometimes silly or even sensual. His lips moved and it appeared as though he was trying to talk to me, as if we actually could communicate with each other. Then, suddenly and unexpectedly, as if with a bolt of invisible lightning, the statue became transformed into a solid-gold, impressively regal sacred treasure, surrounded by filigree of purest gold in intricately beautiful patterns and studded with sparkling diamonds, rubies, sapphires, and emeralds of unquestioned genuineness and value. I registered an impulse to humbly and respectfully bow my head in its presence. If this object existed in the everyday world, there was no question that the Metropolitan Museum of Art in New York would consider it a real find and present it in a well-guarded glass display case.

At the time, amazed though I was at how I had experienced such a transformation of perception and how strikingly beautiful the vision had become, in my report I speculated about projection and transference, assuming that something in my own personal psychodynamics was being expressed and worked out in the movements of the mushroom god. Maybe it was reflecting something of my own sensuality. I imagined how so-called primitive Indians might have claimed that they saw their god, called Teonanácatyl, come alive, perhaps while looking at such a sculpture by firelight after consuming their sacred mushrooms in a religious ceremony. Only now, fifty years later, can I even begin to consider the possibility that the Mazatec god, Teonanácatyl, might actually have been revealed to me. Now I might finally be ready to respect the reality of other experiential worlds and humbly hear and consider whatever he might have to say.

THE ROSE AS AN ARCHETYPE

The rose, especially in the form of a bud with many petals, just starting to open, often appears to have been viewed as a classic, and perhaps universal, symbol of beauty. In psychedelic research, it also manifests as a symbol of the self or of one's own life.

Early psychiatric researchers in Saskatchewan such as Colin Smith, Duncan Blewett, and Nicholas Cwelos, who were investigating the promise of mystical experiences facilitated by LSD in the treatment of alcoholism in the late 1950s, began the tradition of having a single red rose present in the treatment room whenever a psychedelic substance was administered, often accompanied by a little asparagus fern. Practically, it provides a useful point on which to focus attention when one is reorienting oneself from the inner world to the outer world of environmental perceptions, especially when one first sits up and opens one's eyes with eyeshade and headphones removed during a psychedelic session, often prior to a trip to the bathroom. At such times, one would be encouraged to simply "be with the rose" and, if it felt right, to "dive into it" in one's unfolding awareness.

This tradition was continued in research at Spring Grove and has been followed at Johns Hopkins, as well as at most other sites, past and present. As described in the section on External Unity in chapter 5, exquisitely beautiful and meaningful perceptual transformations are often described as research volunteers allow themselves to meditate on the rose. In addition, a visual transformation, frequently and quite reliably, is reported by persons in treatment for addictions, notably for alcoholism. When a volunteer would look at the rose and think about relapsing, he would report visionary changes in which the rose dried up, lost its color, bent over, and died. Conversely, when he focused on the rose with thoughts of sobriety, it would be seen as beautifully unfolding, as in time-lapse photography, a visionary sequence that sometimes would culminate in the external unity of mystical consciousness. Naturally, there is always room for individualized responses; I recall one alcoholic who kissed the rose and then tenderly closed his mouth around it.

Perhaps the equivalent of the rose in Eastern cultures is the lotus flower, sometimes pictured with thousands of unfolding petals. One thinks of the classic Tibetan Buddhist chant "om mani padme hum," roughly translated as "homage to the jewel in the center of the lotus." Many believe that awaiting us all in the vortex of light deep within the jewel is mystical consciousness.

VISIONS AND RELIGIOUS LEADERSHIP

Visionary experiences typically not only are quite amazing to look at, but often carry with them an impetus toward meaningful action, sometimes facilitating changes in both attitudes and behavior. Whether the experience of Moses beholding the burning bush that was not consumed should be viewed as a historical example of external unity (as was suggested by the psychologist of religion Walter Houston Clark) or as a vision without unitive content, the scripture in Exodus (the second book of the Torah) suggests noetic content: "God said to Moses, 'I am who I am'" (Exod. 3:14). The vision is understood to have inspired Moses to lead the Israelites out of bondage in Egypt toward new life in the Land of Canaan. Whether the vision was a pure gift of grace, of God breaking into or manifesting within the consciousness of Moses, or whether the experience was in part made more likely by such factors as personal stress, diet, sleep deprivation, or even by the particular mushrooms Moses might have munched on as he climbed Mount Horeb that day, we will never know. Scholars even debate whether Moses ever existed as a historical personage, or whether he better may be understood as an archetype. It is fascinating to note, however, that Benny Shanon, a professor of psychology at the Hebrew University in Jerusalem, has presented evidence that entheogens found in arid regions of the Sinai Peninsula and the Negev Desert indeed were used for religious purposes by the ancient Israelites. However, it is not how the experience was brought about that mattered, so much as what it meant and what Moses–and perhaps other ancient Israelites–did with it afterward.

Another well-known vision in the scriptures of Judaism, Christianity, and Islam is that of Isaiah in the temple: "I saw the Lord sitting upon a throne, high and lifted up, and his train filled the temple. Above him stood the seraphim: each had six wings: with two he covered his face and with two he covered his feet, and with two he flew. And one called to another and said: 'Holy, holy, holy is the Lord of hosts; the whole earth is full of his glory'" (Isa. 6:1–3). In the scripture, Isaiah responds with fear and guilt, followed by an experience of forgiveness and his acceptance of an invitation to become a prophet, revitalizing the religion of his day.

Central to the birth of early Christianity, of course, is the vision of the Christ on the road to Damascus by Saul of Tarsus. The scriptural account in the Acts of the Apostles reports a flash of light, Saul's question ("Who are you, Lord?"), a convincing experience of the reality of the risen Christ, and a call to become an early missionary. Saul subsequently changed his name to Paul and was transformed from a Roman persecutor of Christians, a man who had allegedly been dragging people out of their homes and imprisoning them for being members of a radical Jewish sect, into a traveling preacher and seminal theologian who wrote the letters to early Christian congregations that now are viewed as sacred books of the New Testament.

ANGELS AND DEMONS

When it comes to angels and demons, probably most of us today think of Renaissance or Baroque art. In our speech we retain references to things angelic and things demonic. Occasionally, some of us, when trying to decide between good and evil (or at least between being fully honest and somewhat devious), may, like medieval monks, imagine a little angel on one shoulder and a little devil on the other, both whispering into our ears. Yet few of us seem to encounter angels and demons very often, or if we do we choose not to share the experiences with most other people. Psychedelic research, however, does suggest that there are heavens and hells within each of us, often populated with fascinating images or beings, and that they are indeed magnificently designed. These visionary entities may be understood as archetypal manifestations that, as in Dante's *Divine Comedy*, dramatically illustrate our psychological processes and spiritual journeys. Often depicted with wings or halos, these beings are found in the literature and art of most world religions, as Muslim or Zoroastrian malaikah, as Buddhist celestial beings called devas, and in Judeo-Christian iconography.

In the Middle Ages, monks may have learned to deal with demons by looking them straight in the eye and holding an elevated cross between themselves and their visions. Similarly, in navigating through the alternative states of consciousness facilitated by entheogens, the intent to confront any visionary manifestation that appears threatening has proved to be of fundamental importance in avoiding panic and in facilitating insight and the resolution of conflicts. Thus, should one encounter a visionary demon, dragon, monster, or bogeyman, one, if well prepared, will steadily and intentionally move toward the manifestation with eye contact if possible, essentially saying, "Hello. Are you ever scary! Why are you here? What are you made of? What might I learn from you?" This is one of those points in a session when the volunteer might reach out for support and interpersonal grounding by holding the hand of a guide or another human being.

Reliably, when this occurs, the image discloses its meaning, which sometimes may trigger screams or tears, often followed by laughter and deep relaxation. The monster sometimes becomes recognized as the abusive babysitter or the angry, alcoholic father, as an expression of one's own shameful past behavior, or even as a symbolic manifestation of some particular fear that one has been avoiding. What is so important here is the discovery that the monster has meaning and in itself is an invitation to enhanced psychological health and spiritual maturation. Its purpose is not to torment, but to teach. That bears repeating: *its purpose is not to torment but to teach!*

With this intention to confront and learn, in the final analysis, it appears that there truly is nothing for one to fear. This makes possible genuine experiences of personality integration and inner peace. Variations on this theme include the insight of a cancer patient in the documentary film *A New Understanding: The Science of Psilocybin*, released in 2014, who discovered that the purpose of the frightening masks he experienced during his psilocybin session was to "scare the fear out of me." Similarly, the role of the huge, imposing black guardian deities who guard the four gates of many classical Tibetan mandalas has been discovered to be protection, ensuring the safety of the meditating pilgrim who dares to venture through the gates and move even more deeply toward the central core of human consciousness.

In this context, as stated earlier, it is understandable why the South American religions that employ ayahuasca in their religious services refer to their sacrament as "the teacher," as do the American Indians who revere peyote. Those who accept the ayahuasca sacrament have received preparation and know, for example, that, should they encounter the great visionary anaconda serpent, they should dive into its mouth and look out through its eyes. This transformational process also illustrates well the potency of one's intention during the alternative states of consciousness facilitated by psychedelic substances. Exploration of consciousness is serious business and the intent to learn and to grow personally and spiritually appears to be critical if safety and benefit are desired. The intent to merely "get high" or "have fun" entails definite risks. My own image for such unwise use of entheogens is playing marbles with diamonds.

In illustration, consider this description from the LSD experience of a middle-aged woman in therapy for a writer's block who also happened to be a scholar of Dante's *Divine Comedy*:

> I am rolling down the circles of hell at a terrifying speed, and this experience overwhelms the others: I am standing by a crib and see through the slats this giant baby face. It is red, screaming, choking on its own spit, covered with mucus. What a terrifying sight an angry baby is to a small child! I must be three years old and I am watching my baby sister. A part of me is very pleased to realize that nobody loves that baby, that nobody wants it. Another part of me is appalled at the baby's pain and cannot bear it. I have the feeling that at this point I am screaming at the

top of my voice, "Please help the baby. Someone please help the baby!" . . . I realize that the baby is not only my sister, but also myself. I was also abandoned when I was that age and left alone to cry like this baby. But about the sister baby, I know that my father and mother now love me, that they don't love the baby. In fact, they hate the baby. I am delighted with this knowledge but also crushed by unbearable guilt. . . . I feel I will suffocate; I will die from the weight of this guilt. The sensations of guilt and rage are so intense and yet such opposites: I feel like I am imploding (constricting, crushed) with guilt and exploding (bursting out, splattering) with rage . . . At this moment guilt and rage dissolve into a hiatus–the silence before the storm.

Vaguely I discern that my sisters and I are three eggs in a nest. I know exactly what it is like to be an egg: I perceive it from outside like a scientist looking through a microscope awed by the miraculous mechanism of life, and from inside as the pulse within the egg. I am the pulse of life and all its endless possibilities. Being an egg is an ecstatic thing; sounds, colors, tastes are all one stupendous pulse but in a brittle shell. I vaguely perceive the nest as being in the pit of hell. . . .

Now takes place the Crux experience of the entire session. I hear the flapping of the devil's giant wings and looking up see the one who laid these eggs. She is a gigantic vulture, as big as the whole infernal sky; she is evil incarnate and she rules the universe. She is zeroing down on us, her little eggs, to destroy us. She is a spectacularly beautiful black vulture: black but very stylized with geometric lines (like an Aztec god), harsh and invulnerable, an invincible force, flapping her black wings like Satan in Dore's illustrations. I realize the little egg nest is hers and so is the pit of hell. The claws are coming down on us to crush us, giant, monstrous claws–and, as I realize that we will be obliterated, an extraordinary revelation takes place. I am filled with horror and relief at the revelation. I am the prophet of the past and the seer of the future and, as I shout my words, I feel that the whole universe shakes with the impact of my truth. Sidereal winds carry my message throughout the galaxies: *My mother is a monster; my mother is a monster.*

But, miraculously, as soon as I scream this, the terrifying vulture splits into a thousand little vultures just as small and helpless as us three little chicks in our eggs. I am overwhelmed by pity and compassion and I see how painful and helpless the vulture's own life has been. In the wonderful literal/figurative manner of LSD, I realize, "How rotten my mother's life has been!," I actually pass through the rot of a vulture's life. I taste the carrion and know experientially how awful it is to be one of the shit-eaters of the world: vultures, villains, and vermin. How rotten are the lives of those who have inflicted pain on others. At this moment, I am filled with compassion and I speak out, not scream, *"poor, poor monster."*

As soon as I say this, or feel this, an extraordinary thing happens: my whole body rises through several layers of ecstatic blue light. I am lying down with my hands across my chest as if I were dead; but instead I am being transported, lifted by angels higher and higher. I am suffused with the most intense feelings of tenderness and love, and know that I have passed from hell into heaven and that this is *divine absolution.* The concept of divine absolution is intensely real and clear. I know that as soon as I forgave my mother monster, God forgave me for hating the baby. The beauty and ecstasy of this moment are indescribable. I realize here that, yes, there are words to describe hell; but none, none at all, for heaven. Every word on this paper is trite, absurd, ridiculous when it tries to express the ecstasy of divine absolution.

PRECIOUS GEMSTONES

Another archetypal manifestation frequently encountered in the visionary world is precious gemstones and metals. The image of the multifaceted diamond of the Self, radiating light and wisdom, is found in religious mystical writings, both Eastern and Western. The descriptions of heaven in the last book of the Christian Bible, the Revelation of John, are familiar to many, complete with streets of gold and gates studded with precious stones, along with majestic thrones, angels, and dragons. As with visionary transformations, such as the mushroom stone described earlier, one cannot help but ask where these amazing experiences come from. Aldous Huxley addressed this question in his essay "Why Are Precious Stones Precious?" He theorized that we value these sparkling little crystals and give them to one another in weddings and on other special occasions as symbols of love, precisely because they remind us of the archetypal gemstones that are innately, perhaps genetically, present within each of our minds. Some would see the light sparkling within them as intrinsically sacred.

MANSIONS OF THE SOUL

Similarly, one can ponder whether the architects in the Middle Ages who constructed Gothic cathedrals with soaring arches and richly hued rose windows or Islamic domes with intricately beautiful patterns and mirrors may actually have been attempting to construct the visionary world in the everyday world of time and space. Visionary imagery of vast architectural spaces is occasionally reported, including the following from the beginning of an experience facilitated by ayahuasca:

Onset was signified by rainbow-hued lines and patterns against a jet black background. Lines were of all colors, one color merging into another through degrees of brightness and saturation, of light and dark, yellow morphing into orange, orange into red, etc. The colors glowed from within, sometimes were iridescent, and at times already appeared alive.

Soon there were architectural visions, initially of the interior of a vast palace (cathedral, office building–whatever you like). There was focused detail of incredibly ornate ceilings and wall panels, often gold designs against a Prussian blue or deep red background with intricate and complex moldings and designs. I noted that this was a form of décor I usually wouldn't find especially interesting or beautiful, though I would have admired the craftsmanship and patient skill required in design and construction. Yet, one vast space would open into another and then yet another and another and another, higher, deeper, wider. These became recognized as the mansions of the soul; I registered the scriptural phase, "In my father's house are many mansions." I recall no furnishings or people, simply the vast, flowing spaces themselves, filled with light and architectural details.

How might we understand an experience like this? Is this a part of heaven, at least one way in which the mind might depict it? The ever-changing perspectives from chamber to chamber were described as akin to the views of a spirit or bird flying somewhere near the arches of the ceilings, Romanesque in this example rather than the more commonly reported Gothic. Whence the light and the intrinsic feeling of sacredness? If a monk encountered a similar experience during deep meditation, it would certainly have seemed reasonable for him to conclude that he had been granted a brief visit to the heavenly realms of the eternal world and might well have called it the Holy City or New Jerusalem.

Perhaps the ancient Hebrew who wrote the eighty-fourth Psalm may have experienced something similar, expressed in the verse, "How lovely is Thy dwelling place, O Lord of Hosts! My soul longs, yea faints for the courts of the Lord; my heart and flesh sing for joy to the living God." Though sometimes interpreted as a song, conceivably by King David, perhaps recalling a visit to the Temple of Solomon in ancient Jerusalem, it could also reflect the vivid memory of a visionary temple, composed by an unknown poet on a Palestinian hillside. Whether his visions may have been facilitated by sacred mushrooms or whether their occurrence was triggered by other means, we will never know. Perhaps they simply happened spontaneously due to divine grace or this psalmist's own unique biochemistry. Many people continue to find his words inspiring and expressive of their own personal devotion.

Various filmmakers, with varying degrees of effectiveness, have attempted to visually portray this experience of steady, progressive movement from one beautiful chamber to another, and another, and another, and yet another, until culmination may occur in the white light of the Void or a similarly ecstatic peak of awareness. Perhaps what is being experienced somehow entails the movement of focused attention from neuron to neuron to neuron. The movement through fractals presented by Simon Powell in his film *Manna–Psilocybin Inspired Documentary* is among the finest I have encountered to date.

THE NATURE AND PROFUNDITY OF MYTH

Archetypes in psychedelic experiences are often encountered within unfolding stories or dramas. Our minds seem to have the ability to create dramas, ingeniously designed, that depict the resolution of our personal conflicts in the context of our spiritual journeys, much like the literary classics *Pilgrim's Progress* by John Bunyan, *The Divine Comedy* by Dante Alighieri, or *Paradise Lost* by John Milton. Volunteers report finding themselves in a particular landscape, whether in medieval Europe or ancient Egypt, or in primeval forests or futuristic cities, in which paths are followed, people and animals are encountered, treasures are discovered, and emotionally potent and insightful experiences occur. Several of our volunteers at Johns Hopkins have reported riding on the back of a huge bird, safely nestled within its feathers, without knowing anything about Garuda, the mythic bird well known in Hinduism and Buddhism. So-called guardian figures, avian, animal, gnome-like, or human, frequently appear early in some psychedelic sessions, seeming to say, "Follow me and I'll lead you where you need to go." Not infrequently, wild or domestic animals appear as supportive companions and teachers.

Sometimes the mind spontaneously produces images of integration following mystical consciousness. For example, I recall the image of the United Nations Building in Manhattan with the colorful flags of the nations of the world on the plaza in front of it. Suddenly the separate colors of each flag flowed into one another to generate a rainbow that arched high over the building. This manifested as a summarizing image at the end of an experience with the entheogen dipropyltryptamine (DPT), the effects of which tend to terminate quite abruptly and completely. One cannot help but feel awe at the creativity within consciousness that produces such images.

When I have finished preparing a person for an experience with an entheogen, usually scheduled for the following day, I often imagine that the person's own mind has composed an opera, perhaps in three acts, and can't wait for the volunteer to experience it. On the next day, of course, the person not only will view the opera with its unique story line, scenery changes, and lighting, but will discover himself or herself in stage center and fully experience it. What is striking is that these experiences do not only occur in people with advanced degrees in literature or creative writing; they routinely occur in the minds of very ordinary people, some of whom have never even attended a college.

The scholarly word for this process of unfolding stories that depict our psychodynamic processes and spiritual quests is *myth*. Joseph Campbell, one of the great scholars of mythology, titled his first book *The Hero with a Thousand Faces*. Each of us, he suggested, is a potential hero on a symbolic journey, and one of the faces is therefore yours and one is mine. In contradistinction to the meaning of "myth" in everyday speech, referring to something that is fabricated or false, real myth is profoundly true.

A VISION OF THE CHRIST

In illustration, here is an example of an encounter with the Christ from the report of a woman minister who received LSD, written in a poetic style:

Vastness. Incredible luminescent light. A different, radiant quality here, never seen before. Filled all space. Exquisite. Beyond description. Unforgettable. Magnificent power–friendly power. Then moments of flames of fire. Indestructible fire. Like Moses' unconsumed burning bush. I could have walked through these friendly flames unharmed. Magnificent light.

Oneness. All one. In-Godness. Indescribable. Utmost. Emotionless. No self. No Sensations. Self was within and without. Time gone. Space gone. Nowhere, but infinitely everywhere. No time, but eternally now. No wholly other or beyond but in it. IN the infinite. In the eternal and infinite. In mystery. Part of it. All one. This seemed an eternity or in no time.

Could see God's view of humanity. Watching mankind destroy itself. Felt helpless to stop it. Utmost love and pity and compassion for all those suffering souls unable to see beyond their own senses, their feelings, their lusts and desires, their machines of destruction, their wars, hates and jealousies, their bodies, their five little senses. Profound love.

Then a magnificent vision of Christ standing motionless in resplendent, radiant Beauty. He had form, but I could almost see through Him; yet I was not really seeing. There was immeasurable power, love. I love Him with a profundity beyond description. I did not walk to Him but was "there"–space and time meaning- less. I was bodyless, selfless. Yet I could grasp His feet and ankles.

I embraced this formless form with an infinite love. Friendly power and love filled the Light. Beyond words. Unforgettable. A slow shifting back to the sense of being In-God and In-Christ. They and I merged, then became separate. It makes sense out of the idea of the Trinity–three in one, separate yet one, per- son and non-person. A most deep understanding of the mean- ing of God giving his Son to this suffering world. I moved into His love-suffering and felt the cost of His life. I took on all the pain of the world, not in general, but person by person, infinitely, all mankind at once. A universal sense of the purpose of the crucifixion–the meaning, the tragedy, the profound love and pity of suffering humanity.

This excerpt from the minister's personal written report of her LSD experience, included in Ralph Metzner's collection of different psychedelic sessions *The Ecstatic Adventure*, clearly appears similar to the historical writings of some of the great Christian mystics, such as St. Teresa of Avila, St. John of the Cross, and Meister Eckhart. One can also speculate that, in the visions of the Christ in the early Christian community, a small Jewish sect at the time, persecuted and meeting in secret, a similar encounter with the Christ archetype may have been taking place. This phenomenon also invites consideration of one way to understand visions of the Christ described in the New Testament, such as that of Mary Magdalene at the empty tomb, the experience of the disciples, Peter, James, and Matthew on the Mount of Transfiguration, and the description of the Ascension of Jesus into heaven.

Biblical scholars have long struggled with trying to discern how literally or how symbolically to understand different verses of scrip- ture and will probably continue to debate alternative interpretations as long as schools of theology exist. What should be viewed as accurate reporting? What should be understood to be symbolic expressions of meaningful experiences as the basic beliefs of the new religion were being formulated in the decades and centuries after the death of the historical Jesus? The visions of the Christ archetype occurring today in the context of psychedelic research and in the use of entheogens in religious settings by indigenous people certainly merit thoughtful acknowledgment and consideration by contemporary theologians and other scholars of religion.

VISIONS DURING MENTAL ILLNESS

The examples presented in this chapter have all been of transient visionary experiences in the minds of basically healthy people and have usually been reported to be meaningful and facilitative of enhanced psychological and spiritual health. Mental health professionals know well that similar experiences, usually called hallucinations, are also reported by distressed people who are often given the diagnoses of schizophrenia or bipolar disorder and who appear basically unable to take responsibility for their lives amid the flux of their mental experiences. In his own definition of mystical consciousness, William James included a category called "Transiency" (along with "Ineffability," "Noetic Quality," and "Passivity") to emphasize the brief duration of the alternative state of awareness and the subsequent return to normative functioning in the world.

The psychiatrist Loren Mosher, building on the theories of R. D. Laing, believed that some of these people, especially early in the manifestation of their symptoms, could be helped to move through the alternative states they were experiencing toward resolution and healing if sufficient emotional support were made available to them in a treatment facility, such as his Soteria House in San Jose, California, with a staff that emphasized trust, respect, and interpersonal grounding. In psychedelic research, one can easily observe how states of mind characterized by panic, confusion, suspiciousness, and paranoid misinterpretation of the environment and the motives of others can easily become manifested when a solid, respectful relationship between the volunteer and the researcher or guide has not been established in advance. It seems reasonable to assume that similar dynamics may be present when alternative states of consciousness spontaneously occur and, without interpersonal grounding, spiral out of control.

Mosher's proposal remains a controversial and inadequately researched hypothesis. Reliance on current biological psychiatry and antipsychotic medications in an effort to terminate alternative states and rapidly restore the minds of disturbed people to normative baselines has been the dominant treatment modality in the United States in recent years. Perhaps the day will come when a balanced approach will prevail that values both helpful medications and alternative states of awareness.

PART III

Personal and
Interpersonal Dynamics

8

The Interpersonal and the Mystical

As the intuitive choreography of experiential content in psychedelic sessions unfolds, it is often quite amazing to witness how one's relationships with other persons and one's readiness to experience mystical states of awareness are meaningfully interconnected. Martin Buber, a Jewish existentialist philosopher known for his focus on the sacredness of relationships, coined the term "the I-Thou relationship" (from "Ich-Du," employing the more intimate, second-person, singular German pronoun), for relationships both between separate, individual human beings and between each of us and the "Eternal Thou," or God. Many psychedelic experiences appear to validate Buber's theme that the manner in which we interact with one another does really matter in terms of spiritual health and growth.

AT THE GATE BEFORE THE INFINITE ROSE GARDEN

Among the cancer patients I've been able to support during the effects of psychedelic substances, a tall, thin woman I'll call Rosa comes vividly to mind. She was an African American mother of two daughters, had worked hard as a college custodian, and now was coping with the final stages of uterine cancer. At this point in her illness, she had to endure the almost constant vaginal discharge of bodily fluids, so during our preparatory and integrative appointments she sat on a portable toilet with a white blanket discretely placed on her lap. Nonetheless, she welcomed the counseling intervention that had been offered to her in hopes of preparing more fully for her death and perhaps decreasing some of her psychological distress.

After we had spent approximately eight hours together, establishing a trust-filled relationship, she was admitted to a private hospital room for her psychedelic session. There, the nurse assisting me as a cotherapist administered a moderate dose of dipropyltryptamine (DPT) to her. As her experience began, she encountered a rocky landscape through which she had to make her way, coming more fully to terms with her diagnosis and prognosis in the process. Finally, she arrived at a visionary gate, where she could hear the singing of angels and beyond which she reported "roses as far as the eye could see." Just as she was about to step through the gate, she heard (within her own mind) the voice of one of her daughters calling her. Reluctantly, with some irritation, she turned around to "find out what she wanted." Then, to her dismay, she discovered that the alternative states of consciousness were abruptly ending and that once again she was lying without visionary imagery in her hospital bed. She voiced her frustration in the dialect of Baltimore's inner city: "If I *evaah* see that gate again" (pause, followed by loud, rushed speech), "I'm a goin' right on through!"

Back in the everyday world, in the weeks prior to her death, Rosa did interact with this daughter, as well as other family members, manifesting an openness that was new for them. Together they addressed conflicts that had prevailed between them in ways that were profoundly reconciling. This same daughter invited Rosa to come and live with her during the final weeks before nursing home care became imperative. After the eventual transfer to the nursing home had occurred, I happened to arrive for a follow-up visit just moments after Rosa's death, where I encountered her two daughters crying in the entry foyer. When her breathing had become markedly irregular, a very anxious nurse had ordered the daughters out of her room, closed the white curtains around her bed, and left her alone to die. At my insistence, and "only under my supervision," the daughters and I returned to the bedside, viewed Rosa's body, and talked some of how much their relationship had meant.

Subsequently, I received the following letter:

Dear Dr. Richards,

I had never watched anyone dying before. Thank you for giving me the chance to say and do so many things for my mother, that others like me never had the chance to do for theirs . . . I'm still grieving for my mother. Maybe I'm grieving and crying for all the wasted times in our lives. I was the black sheep in my family, but in the end I had a place for my mother to come and stay. We became very good friends in the end. We both asked each other's forgiveness and we both gave it. My mother asked me not to be sad or afraid of her when she died. Thank you for telling me that the only way to conquer your fears is to face them; I didn't know that. Out of all the sadness and pain, something good came out of it.

Although we have no way of knowing exactly what Rosa may have experienced as her death occurred, it is reasonable for me to imagine that she indeed went through the visionary gate and danced through the fields of roses and beyond while angels sang.

THE EMERALD ON THE VELVET PILLOW

Another illustration of the role of interpersonal relationships in psychedelic sessions comes from an experience facilitated by DPT of a middle-aged woman I will call Cora. Struggling with terminal breast cancer, this African American social worker was struggling with accepting the imminence of her death and leaving her husband and two sons who were in early adulthood.

As the effects of DPT began, Cora discovered a vision of a magnificent deep green emerald that was resting on a velvet pillow. During the next few hours, she experienced four approaches to this precious stone. The first time, the focus was on her relationship with her husband. She explored the many facets of their long commitment to each other, said tearfully aloud, "How could you be so many things to me?," and finally accepted that she had to die soon and managed to let go of her desire to cling to him. With this experience of "letting go," she reported a surge of gratitude for the quality of life they had shared.

Then the emerald reappeared and her focus changed to the elder of her two sons and her ambivalence about his intention to marry a woman who already had a child from another relationship. She sorted through her feelings and finally affirmed her acceptance of her son's decision and also of her future daughter-in-law and granddaughter.

The emerald reappeared a third time and her mind presented her with her younger son, who had not excelled academically and who reminded her in some ways of her homosexual brother. Again she struggled through her many feelings until she finally was able to affirm her acceptance of him as he is, regardless of his academic accomplishments or possible sexual preference.

It was at this point, after resolving the emotions connected with her three most primary human relationships, that she approached the emerald a fourth time. This time, she experienced herself being drawn within the crystalline beauty of the gemstone and became immersed in mystical consciousness. Why this particular woman's mind chose an emerald on a velvet pillow as an archetypal symbol of the Self rather than the more common image of a diamond remains unknown. (I do recall another woman who, in an experience facilitated by LSD, found herself entering mystical consciousness through a vision of a yellow topaz.) Perhaps the velvet pillow was a symbol of the approach of death and also the pillow on which her head would rest in her casket. In the wisdom of her mind, her relationships between her husband and two sons clearly had to be addressed before she was ready to experience her relationship with Buber's "Eternal Thou."

The intense quantity of therapeutic work within a period of approximately four hours is striking. There is no way her experience could be viewed merely as "getting high" or as escape from life. The entheogen wisely and powerfully drew her into the primary vortexes of her psychological distress and spiritual life.

THE VEILS IN THE FIREPLACE

Yet another classic example of this apparent wisdom within many, if not all, human minds is the story of the theological student who, while diligently pursuing his graduate studies, had been neglecting his wife and children. In the early days of research in Boston, he took LSD in a living-room setting and, with open eyes, saw many visionary veils superimposed before a fireplace. The veils appeared like curtains between himself and the burning logs. Intuitively, he interpreted them as barriers between himself and God. Slowly, with the expressive movement of his arms, he pulled one veil after the other aside until only one remained. He braced himself for what he was convinced would be "the great experience of seeing the Face of God." Dramatically, he then pulled the last veil aside and found himself almost brutally confronted by a vivid vision of his three children crying for their father.

Though not validated by the usual methods in social science research, it was claimed that the powerful flood of tears he manifested at that point was shared simultaneously by his children at their home in New Hampshire, several hours away. It is also claimed that the experience facilitated a better balance between his roles as scholar, spouse, and parent.

This constitutes another example of how people often tend to experience not what they expect or want, but what they appear to require or need on their particular thresholds of psychological and spiritual development. In similar fashion, I have found myself supporting several Roman Catholic priests who asked to participate in research studies in hopes of glimpsing the mystical state Christians call "the beatific vision." Some, though certainly not all, found themselves painfully sorting through traumatic experiences and issues in their early sexual development instead.

9

Experiences of Meaninglessness, Despair, and Somatic Discomfort

THE POWER OF AN EMOTIONAL BATH

One of the first cancer patients who I guided through psychedelic therapy was a fifty-year-old, Jewish woman we can call Sarah with two children in early adolescence. Her husband, colluding with her surgeon, had decided that she could not cope with the knowledge that her cancer was terminal. He took her on vacation to a Caribbean island where, instead of having a wonderful time, she felt physically weak and in pain, sensed her husband wasn't being fully truthful, and finally broke through his denial. Angry and depressed on her return to Baltimore, she sent her two children off to summer camps without telling them of the seriousness of her condition, hoping to be dead before they returned. She also decided not to tell her elderly mother of her illness, for fear it would "kill her." Her relationships with her husband and mother-in-law were at best perfunctory. Her husband was "such a good man" that he telephoned his mother almost every night just before they climbed into bed together. Her mother-in-law visited most days, usually just prior to her bridge game, so she could report to her partners that she had dutifully looked in on her daughter-in-law.

Sarah dreaded those visits and felt they were inherently phony, but had endured them like a hopeless prisoner.

As preparation for her LSD session proceeded, she described her concept of death as "a lightbulb going out." If life after death made any sense, it was through her good deeds as they manifested in the lives of her children and, someday, her children's children, a perspective often called "social immortality." She had read *The Beyond Within*, written by the psychiatrist Sidney Cohen, a book that described how some cancer patients experienced Van Gogh–like visual transformations during the effects of LSD. So it was that, when she was admitted to Sinai Hospital in Baltimore for her LSD session, she had several valuable paintings and sculptures moved from her home into her private room, hoping to enjoy enhanced aesthetic perceptiveness during her psychedelic session.

The content of her journey within, however, consisted of reliving many years of chronic loneliness and depression, which she summarized as "an emotional bath"–what many would call "a bad trip." She had no interest in looking at the paintings or sculptures in her room while the consciousness-altering effects of LSD were still active. Whether the session included a glimpse of mystical consciousness or not, I could not determine; the only positive experience she would describe was a scene as she was returning to normal of bouncing yellow balls in the streets of Manhattan, reminding her of a happy experience she once shared there with her sister.

When the effects of LSD were subsiding, her husband, mother-in-law, sister, and a close friend were invited to enter her room to visit her. They cautiously assembled around her hospital bed. When her mother-in-law bent over to give her a kiss, Sarah yanked off the woman's wig and then sat up regally in bed, pausing dramatically, and then saying, "It is true that I am dying, but let's get something straight. I am not dead yet!" (The last three words were spoken slowly and deliberately with seething intensity.) The "emotional bath" rapidly became a shared experience for everyone present.

Returning home, she summoned her children from their summer camps, one at a time, and personally prepared them for her death. She did the same with her mother and was relieved to discover that her mother "rose to the occasion" and did not die. She expressed anger at her husband and mother-in-law for having misjudged her capacity to cope with her situation and told off her surgeon, and those relationships all came alive in new ways. She enjoyed visiting with friends and giving away selected pieces of jewelry to them.

On the day prior to her death, as Sarah was on the verge of becoming comatose, I visited her, once again in a hospital room. She expressed appreciation for the benefit she had experienced, and also a sense of awe at the potential import of the research we were conducting. I asked her if she still thought death would be "like a lightbulb going out." She smiled, looked me in the eye, and softly yet firmly said, "Yes." Then she paused and added, "But I'm willing to be surprised." She pointed to her lips and requested a goodbye kiss. I left her with her sister, who held her hand as she slid into deepening coma and died.

So, what happened here? If she experienced any mystical glimpses, she chose not to share them or perhaps lacked the vocabulary to speak of them. It appears that several long hours of crying and reliving a life history of feeling lonely and chronically depressed in a supportive atmosphere with an abundance of interpersonal acceptance proved to be profoundly therapeutic for her. Was hers a "bad trip"? I think not. As expressed by others, she appeared to have experienced "not what she wanted, but what she needed."

A BRIEF INTRODUCTION TO PSYCHOSIS

Nearing the end of my studies in Germany and not knowing if I ever would have a legal opportunity to take a psychedelic substance again after my return to the United States, I asked Dr. Leuner if I could have one final psychedelic adventure in his clinic. He was happy to provide whatever substance and dose I requested, but felt he was too busy to personally monitor the session. Walter Pahnke had left Göttingen at this point to visit a center where psychedelic research was progressing in Italy. Thus, I had to locate someone else to spend the day with me. Doubting that I really needed anyone anyway, I approached the one other American theology student at the university and proceeded to give him a brief lesson on how to be a supportive guide. I then opted to receive a very high dose of psilocybin (40 mg of regular psilocybin, called C-39, in liquid form, administered intramuscularly in two injections).

Both the friend I had enlisted to support me and I proved totally unprepared to deal with the states of consciousness that occurred. I subsequently described my experience as "hanging onto a rope behind a jet plane." Though I expected to be capable of trusting and "letting go" as I had during prior experiences, this time it appears that I involuntarily "held on" with a sense of desperation. I experienced what I subsequently called a "toxic psychosis," with involuntary muscular discharges, profuse sweating, and blatant paranoia. Suddenly it was clear to me that the patients in the hallway were obviously Secret Service agents and I wondered how I could have been so naïve as not to have recognized that sooner. Dr. Leuner in Germany and Dr. Leary in the United States clearly were in cahoots with each other in a plot to alter the course of civilization as both of their names started with the letter L. But of greatest concern, there was no order, no symmetry, no beauty, nothing that felt of religious import. The state was clearly "beyond time" and could well be called "cosmic."

In my report, I wrote, "The memory that I had once lived on earth, had been born of human parents and nurtured in human society seemed little more than a curious memento or a mythical tale of questionable validity. So it was that the most concrete things to which I could relate in order to find some footing in this realm were the most abstract of philosophical categories." At one point, I became convinced that I had died and was being initiated into some form of an afterlife, and felt intense regret at the inconvenience and professional embarrassment I had caused Dr. Leuner. He had allowed me to have this final psilocybin experience out of the goodness of his heart; now he had to report an "adverse reaction" to the university and government authorities and ship my body back to the United States. Then, suddenly all this chaos ceased and, after a period of exhausted silence, I found that my everyday self had reconstituted itself and, surprisingly, that I again was well oriented and energized and seemed able to think with exceptional clarity.

Was this a "bad trip"? I answer in the affirmative. Though I acquired some experiential learning, notably about how paranoia develops when one is unable to trust and needs to maintain control and how there are alternative states of consciousness devoid of beauty or meaning, the experience was not therapeutic, inspiring, or life-enhancing. Perhaps I learned some humility. Perhaps I experienced a chastening correction to my enthusiasm and acquired increased awareness of the potential of psychedelic drugs to negatively impact people's lives when they are administered without sufficient knowledge or skill.

Ever since, I have emphasized the importance of interpersonal grounding, that is, having someone present who one honestly can choose to trust without reservation. The attitude "I can manage on my own and don't really need anyone else" clearly can be very counterproductive in some high-dose sessions when the "I" needs to totally relinquish control. It has seemed to me that there is something within our minds that requires acknowledgment of our interconnectedness with and dependence upon other people in everyday life, at least on some occasions, before the doors to eternal realms of awareness can fully open. To this day, I attribute this chaotic learning experience both to an inadequately established relationship with a guide and to dosage that, at least for me at that time, was too high. Interesting enough, it has never caused me to question the validity of the mystical states of consciousness that occurred in my life prior to this experience or that have recurred since that time.

DISCOVERING MEANING IN PSYCHOSOMATIC DISTRESS

An example of physical, psychosomatic discomfort is illustrated in the following report from an experience facilitated by psilocybin. This volunteer, a man suffering from anxiety symptoms secondary to prostate cancer, had also suffered from Perthes in childhood, a disease of the hip joint that over the years had caused significant physical and emotional pain in his life. His description, excerpted from his psilocybin session report, follows:

> At some point, my left knee began to twitch and shake. This is the knee that was first operated on when I was eight years old, then again when I was twelve, and finally replaced with an artificial knee implant. . . . This twitching is something I've experienced many times, even before the replacement surgery, mostly at night

when I'm sleeping. . . . The twitching is often accompanied by a deep ache and sensation of cold in my knee. I've often thought this was a psychosomatic response since my knee is plastic and metal and has no nerve endings to experience pain or cold . . .

During the session, the knee movement came to dominate everything. My whole body kept shifting, trying to find respite. For what seemed like hours, I writhed and sweated on the couch, unable to find relief. A lot of this period is a blur. The guides talked to me and I remember my hand being held. Though I can't recall this episode in detail, I know that this was a key episode of the session. I came to fully realize, for the first time, that the surgeries on my left knee, especially the two during childhood, were deeply traumatizing. I also realized that my subconscious wanted me to know this. Of all the things the psilocybin experience could have shown me–visions of the unity of life, soaring into the heavens, seeing lost loved ones–it was the lifelong burden of unresolved trauma that was revealed.

The horrible thing about surgery is you're medicated so your conscious brain forgets the experience, but your subconscious mind and your body know what's happening. The most apt way I can think to express this is to use the title from a science fiction story I once read–"I Have No Mouth and I Must Scream." . . . When my knee has ached in the past, whether the real bony structure or the metal-and-plastic replacement, I was often angry and would curse my knee and the pain. Now I realize that my knee bore great suffering and, for much of my life, carried my body weight when I was standing in order to protect my right hip. My conscious self believed that the Perthes disease of my right hip was my defining childhood trauma. Using crutches and wearing a leg-sling to keep my right leg from touching the ground and then, later, wearing a full-length weight-bearing brace on that leg–all this happened from ages five to fifteen and dominated my world view. My left, normal, leg was there to carry my weight, there to protect my right leg, there to be cut open and have metal pins inserted to stunt its growth so that my right leg, whose growth was slowed because of the Perthes, wouldn't be freakishly short compared to the left.

In my session with psilocybin, I came to realize that my left leg has steadfastly supported me while suffering greatly. My subconscious, until now, has never been able to adequately express that pain. Interestingly, when I was four years old, I first began to have symptoms of Perthes, which manifested itself as pain in the knees. My mother took me to a series of doctors who all diagnosed my symptoms as growing pains. I also distinctly remember my father telling me that my pain was "all in my head." I'm acutely aware, and have been for much of my life, that my lifelong anger at people who don't believe me when I tell them something or who won't pay attention to what I have to say, goes back to this childhood dismissal about leg pain.

I will continue to work at understanding this revelation about my knee. I already have a different relationship with my knee because I no longer feel anger toward it. There's more to do–perhaps somatic experiencing, massage therapy, meditative practice.

When I reached the end of this part of my psilocybin experience, all my twitching stopped and my knee felt cool and relaxed. It was a wonderful feeling.

Without an understanding of psychosomatic symptoms, ways emotions become manifested in muscular tension, tremors, and pain–or sometimes nausea, cardiovascular symptoms, and headaches–an observer could well have thought this man's discomfort in his legs was simply an adverse reaction to a drug. Entheogens are often called "meaning-making substances," and this is one illustration of the meaning that can be expressed in physical distress symptoms. This volunteer, like others mentioned, essentially said, "I didn't experience what I wanted, but I experienced what I needed." Whereas this man would have preferred a beautiful, spiritual experience of some kind, what he encountered was chronic psychological conflict awaiting insight and resolution. In the report of his second psilocybin session, which due to the research protocol happened to be in low dosage, he summarized what he had learned:

I reflected on the difficulty I have in trusting others, something I know goes back to my childhood with an unreliable alcoholic father. . . . I realized that the hard work of the first psilocybin session was the result of a massive discharge of negative energy from childhood trauma involving my left knee. I also realized that I'd blamed my left knee for a lifetime of pain but the psilocybin experience helped me see that my knee, though it had been severely traumatized, had still held up me, still supported me all these years. . . . I can see that [my] untrustworthy father and what I considered an untrustworthy body have created the difficulty I continue to struggle with in trusting others. I'm hoping that my experiences and insights gained during the psilocybin treatments will help me make progress in this area.

NAUSEA AND VOMITING

A common psychosomatic manifestation during psychedelic sessions is nausea, generally understood as anxiety manifested in the digestive system. In preparing people for sessions, we instruct them to accept nausea and to "dive into their stomachs" like diving into a swimming pool if it should occur. This often suffices to immediately terminate the symptom and to allow the flow of attention to move elsewhere. Sometimes, however, the nausea is persistent and the person needs to "spit something out" or briefly vomit. This we handle by simply directing the person to sit up for a few moments, providing support to his or her back, speaking a few supportive words, and providing an emesis basin as needed. We then immediately encourage the person to recline again and continue the unfolding journey–typically without even removing the eyeshade or headphones if they are already in place.

Usually such episodes of vomiting are experienced as cleansing or cathartic, as if one is purifying oneself of emotional garbage, such as fear, grief, guilt, or anger. Nausea is especially common in the psychedelic sessions of people with alcoholic histories, perhaps associated with memories of being drunk and feelings of shame and failure. Vomiting, sometimes combined with diarrhea, called *La Purga*, is also frequently reported to occur in the religious gatherings of those who use ayahuasca as their sacrament and is accepted as healthy purgation and cleansing. Perhaps there are other plant substances than the psychoactive DMT in some of the brews that may increase the probability of nausea. However, it is noteworthy that many people do not vomit at all during the action of either ayahuasca or other psychedelic substances. It appears to be more of a psychogenic manifestation, even an expectation effect, than a reliable physiological response to the sacrament itself. It may be seen as one symbolic way of learning to trust and to fully relinquish control. It may well be that the same principles apply to the religious use of peyote, again where vomiting frequently occurs and is usually viewed as a beneficial response.

The examples in this chapter well illustrate some of the difficult and painful experiences that can occur during psychedelic sessions. Often the pain—physical, psychological, or both—does appear to have a purpose and a meaning, and it often culminates in very positive feelings of freedom and relief and new insights. However, as noted earlier, it makes clear that, if one simply wants delightful escape from the pressures of life, psychedelic substances are very poor choices. Psychological and spiritual growth is indeed serious and sometimes gut-wrenching business.

10

Religious Conversion and Psychodynamic Experiences

VARIETIES OF EXPERIENCES IN REVIVAL SERVICES

Those who have grown up in branches of Christianity with a strong evangelical heritage, or who have visited churches often considered "fundamentalistic," are familiar with the tradition of the altar-call. Typically at the close of a sermon or during the singing of a final hymn, people in attendance are invited, if so moved, to leave their seats, walk to the front of the worship space, and kneel, thereby "becoming saved" or "accepting the Lord Jesus Christ as their personal savior." The clergy and elders present warmly welcome those who come forward, often praying with them or laying hands upon their heads. Some people decisively choose to accept this invitation for the first time; others may participate periodically as a means of renewing their religious commitment. Sometimes this occurs in the context of several consecutive days of services with sermons and music called a revival or a crusade.

If somehow one could enter into the heads of each of the people who chose to come forward or, if in a religious sanctuary, who knelt at the communion rail, and then feel their experiential worlds and look out through their eyes, I suspect that one would discover a rather wide range of states of consciousness. Some probably would have responded out of social pressure alone, would be feeling quite self-conscious and awkward, wouldn't really be sure what to expect, and couldn't wait to escape to the parking lot when the service was over. Some others would have honestly faced up to powerful emotions that they had been avoiding, perhaps "sins" of selfishness, greed, jealousy, or guilt, perhaps coupled with behavior they regretted associated with infidelity or substance abuse problems, and earnestly prayed for forgiveness. They may well have found themselves crying, soaking up the warmth and acceptance of the congregation, and pledging themselves to new forms of behavior more in accordance with the ethical standards of the community. They would have made a courageous and conscious choice to call attention to themselves and, in the privacy of their own minds if not publicly, to confess their distress or perceived moral failings. In kneeling, they would have expressed an openness and a willingness to receive that in many ways parallel the decision to trust and the subsequent passive receptivity critical to the occurrence of constructive experiences during the action of psychedelic substances.

Some of those tearful people standing or kneeling in front of the assembled congregation might have been experiencing confession and social acceptance alone, perhaps within a belief system of "accepting Jesus." Occasionally, however, some may also have been experiencing visionary or archetypal states of mind, perhaps accompanied by a convincing sense of a loving presence, sometimes identified as the eternal Christ, with or without actual visionary imagery. On rare occasions, mystical consciousness as defined in this book may have been encountered, complete with noetic insights and a convincing awareness of the reality of an eternal dimension. For most who experienced intense catharsis, the support of the people assembled would have been sufficient to have enabled them to leave the service with feelings of new hope and gratitude, fully capable of driving home safely. A few may have expressed more emotion than adequately could be processed within the available time, and may have needed continuing support, with or without formal mental health care.

PSYCHOLYTIC, PSYCHEDELIC,
AND PSYCHODELYTIC THERAPY

Similarly, during the action of entheogens, there are usually a variety of states of consciousness, some of which may focus on personal emotions and memories without explicit religious content. When entheogens have been administered in attempts to deepen and accelerate psychotherapy, often in repetitive low dosages, the content of sessions often includes the reliving of traumatic childhood experiences and the sorting out of emotions of guilt, fear, anger, and grief. Here, instead of the presence of the minister and congregation, the acceptance and steady presence of the psychotherapist or guide provide the interpersonal grounding requisite for healing. Especially in Europe, psychedelic substances were used in mental health clinics in this manner, often labeled as psycholytic (mind-releasing) therapy.

A Dutch psychiatrist, G. W. Arendsen-Hein, integrated the psycholytic approach with the higher-dosage psychedelic form of treatment in a clinic known as Veluweland that he designed in Ederveen, a suburb of Amsterdam. There he administered a series of low-dose sessions, once or twice a week, to his patients (registered as "guests") in small rooms until he judged that they had adequately addressed their personal, psychodynamic issues. Then he would admit them into a beautifully designed, significantly larger room, often for a single high-dose session, in hopes of facilitating a mystical type of experience. As I recall his psychedelic room, the green carpet merged with the green grass outside a large picture window, where one might well see swans gliding on a small pond. Within the room were comfortable furnishings, a fireplace, and a sculpture of the Buddha. Arendsen-Hein posited that the most effective treatment included both sessions that focused on what Carl Jung called the "personal unconscious" and a mystical encounter with the "collective unconscious" that was believed to provide a profound sense of integration and a deeper feeling of being at home in the world. Unfortunately, like most of the clinicians who used psychedelic substances with their patients in the 1960s, Arendsen-Hein had neither the resources nor the inclination to pursue carefully designed research protocols with control groups that today are expected in the scientific community in order to establish the effectiveness of a new treatment modality.

In the use of psychedelic substances in psychotherapy, there are clearly two potential trajectories, both of which appear to work well. In one, the person gradually works through personal psychodynamic experiences en route to the realm of transcendental forms of consciousness. This approach is most congruent with psychoanalytic approaches to treatment. In the other, which uses higher dosage, it may be possible for some people to experience mystical and archetypal forms of consciousness in an initial session, sometimes sort of making an end-run around any personal conflicts that might eventually need to be addressed. Then, in the weeks and months afterward, in light of the memory of mystical consciousness, one addresses the issues of personal, psychodynamic import. This approach appears to work especially well with people suffering from addictive disorders, who have lived with an abundance of low self-worth, fueled by repetitive experiences of failure and shame. For them the shift in self-concept facilitated by an initial glimpse of mystical consciousness, in which they discover undeniable beauty, worth, and positive resources within their minds, appears to make it more easy to subsequently confront the abundance of negative emotions and memories within.

The following excerpt from the report of the high-dose LSD session of a man who had been addicted to narcotic drugs, imprisoned, and paroled to a halfway house for treatment in one of the research studies conducted at the Maryland Psychiatric Research Center illustrates well how the insights of mystical consciousness can flow into human relationships:

> It is really hard to put into words what I really experienced in my session. I don't think there are words to express all the beauty I saw and felt. I began to flow with the music. It seemed as though I became the music and the music became me. We became one and the journey on to a universe which is full of love and divine beauty began. . . . I saw a Divine Being before me who had His hand out and stood alone and glowing with a radiance of love, beauty, faith, and trust. My mind left my body and my body was dead. As I touched His hands, I became Him or we become one. . . .

I knew then that I had all these within me: beauty, faith, love, and trust. I had touched that Divine Being and became part of God. At that moment, I shouted: "Good God Almighty, what a beautiful day! Great God Almighty, I am a man at last!" . . . I have been cleansed of all my sins. I thought before this moment that I could see but I have been a blind man all my life.

Then I saw [my wife] and my kids and it seemed as if she and I went into each other's arms as one. . . . Then I could see all the wrong and unhappiness I had caused her and the children. . . . I experienced all the wrong deeds I had done in life and I truly believe that I have been forgiven. . . .

I became more aware of my blackness. I am proud that I am of black heritage. But black or white, under our skin we are all the same; we are all brothers and children of God. Through my experience, I know that I'll never use drugs again or turn back to the slick way of life.

Another illustration comes from the report of a man being treated for alcoholism with DPT-assisted psychotherapy who encountered more struggle in letting go of usual control:

The experience began not long after receiving the injection and it seemed right away like I got into a battle of sorts, like I guess with demons and devils, and whatever. This seemed to last for quite a while and then we'd be transported into another world and kind of go from one world to another. It seemed pretty far out. There was a whole range of emotions from a lot of fear, from fear to anger to love to beauty to contentment to the fullest extent possible, I believe. At times it came to panic and became paranoid at one point, when I began to think there was a plot to steal my identity, to steal my soul, and even [my therapist and cotherapist] were in on it and I wasn't sure. I was trying to hold on to reality. I wanted to make sure I would come back to reality but then I kept getting taken in different worlds. Time meant nothing and space really meant nothing and what was real and what wasn't real became really confused. . . . I remember then at that point I seemed to be searching for who I was, who Sam Jones [pseudonym] was, and trying to find him, what he was like.

I'd go back into the past and I kept getting in touch with the past, like the eighteenth century, seventeenth century, the time of the Crusades. I kept going back there from time to time. At one point, it seemed like I was in the Far East, in China or some place and I was trying to talk in an Asian tongue, some Asian dialect. I was trying to mutter and talk in that dialect. Then I would go off again up into some dazzling white lights.

One part was like you've known the beauty, the utmost in beauty. The thing about the beauty was the purity of it. It was dazzling and sparkling. I couldn't see anything but that and then we go back and dig out some more monsters, dig out some more demons as it were, and almost do combat in battle with them, an experience of intense fear and panic, and then go back to kind of a warm feeling.

I experienced death, kind of met death, and from death was like transported up into this beauty, into this white light, dazzling brilliance, and then I began to come out of it. . . . I still wasn't sure I was in touch with reality. I was afraid, really at one point. I was afraid I would never get back in touch with reality and that it was all part of a plot and that I would never come back to the world as I know it. I would kind of exist out in the universe as a part of the cosmos and go from one world to another and yet I could see from time to time the people who were real in my world, like my wife and my children. . . .

I experienced the ultimate in feeling of love and as I came out of it, eventually I gradually began to realize I was back on the couch and the panic stopped. I wasn't afraid any more that I'd lose touch with reality. . . . I feel I found out something about myself. I let myself realize that there is goodness in people, and particularly in myself. And I think I found an inner strength that I didn't have before. I kind of looked at myself really for the first time and more or less kind of found out who I was.

11

Discipline and Integration

TIMOTHY LEARY AND THE MILLBROOK ESTATE

Seven grams of Timothy Leary's cremains were launched into outer space, slightly over a year from the date of his death in 1996. Purportedly, they orbited the earth for six years before the Pegasus rocket carrying them burned up in the atmosphere. Many would counsel me to let their remnants and the man they represented remain wherever they may be and not even to mention the "L word." Whether it stands for "Leary" or "LSD," it tends to evoke strongly irrational and stereotypical responses. Some may view him as a charismatic, prophetic hero, far ahead of his time; others see him as an irresponsible, psychologically troubled researcher, who abandoned the disciplines and cautions of science to seek publicity with movie stars and encourage teenagers to break laws and allow their lives to be derailed by the seductive traps of drug abuse. Either way, his name and image have assumed almost archetypal status in many modern minds.

How history will judge him is an open question. In 1963, the construction of William James Hall was completed at Harvard University, a stunningly attractive high-rise building that has become home to the social science departments, designed by Minuoru Yamasaki (the same highly regarded architect who designed the original World Trade towers in New York). Although in his days as a Harvard professor William James made many contributions to psychology and philosophy that are often respectfully acknowledged by current scholars, he also explored alternative states of consciousness with nitrous oxide gas and openly wrote about his experiences. Whether or not Harvard will ever erect a building or even install a modest sculpture in the shaded corner of a quadrangle in honor of Timothy Leary remains to be seen. President Nixon's description of him as "the most dangerous man in America" still reverberates in many minds.

While studying in Germany and encountering my first psychedelic experiences in 1963 and 1964, I read about Timothy Leary, Richard Alpert, and Ralph Metzner in *Time* magazine, along with news of the "Harvard scandal." I was not sure what to make of this controversy in the United States, as research with psychedelic drugs in Europe was progressing without fanfare in reasonable, academically respectable ways. Nonetheless, I decided I wanted to meet these men, collect my own impressions, and make my own decisions. So it was that, on the day of my return to the United States, after my plane from Luxembourg landed at Kennedy Airport, I immediately boarded a train to Millbrook, New York. At that point in time, psychedelic research at Harvard had ceased and Timothy and his colleagues were living on an estate owned by the family of Peggy Hitchcock, an heiress of the Mellon fortune. Having established through prior correspondence that I was welcome, a taxi dropped me at a stone gatehouse similar to the entrance of a European castle.

With a knapsack on my back on a hot August day, I followed a long, curving road toward an impressive, old white mansion with an imposing turret. Someone greeted me, led me up two flights of stairs to a small room with a mattress on the floor, and informed me that Timothy was "swimming at the waterfall with his companion, a Swedish model," but would return soon and that I could hike to the waterfall and join them if I so desired. The idea appealed to my sweaty and weary self, but, as I followed the woodland trail to the waterfall and saw Timothy nude in the distance, I decided to return to the mansion, shower in an ordinary bathroom, and await his return. I needed some time to adjust to a world very different than my life in German academia.

The mansion itself proved to be an intriguing place, full of fascinating architectural details, and occupied by diverse people from different cultural backgrounds and careers, all open to expressing stimulating and potentially innovative ideas. There was a delightful monkey in the kitchen. No one seemed obsessed with order or cleanliness; all was comfortable and casual—or what some would call chaotic and disordered. Meals, incidentally, were quite flavorful and were typically preceded by a period of silence, during which all present were encouraged to attune themselves to gratitude and to focus attention with full sensory openness on appreciating the taste of the first morsel of nourishment.

When Timothy appeared on the day of my arrival, he gave me his full attention, genuinely interested in what had been occurring with Leuner's research in Göttingen and within me as a person. His companion, Nena von Schlebrügge, who became the third of his five wives, impressed me as being as beautiful spiritually as she was physically. When I left a few days later, Timothy personally drove me to the train station and wished me well. We maintained periodic communication and he welcomed me for occasional weekend seminars during the following two years. Many of those seminars were conducted and attended by highly respected scientists and academicians.

It was clear that more was going on at Millbrook than merely some sort of hedonistic, countercultural protest. Along with the seminars and attempts to establish a successful community, I was told of nights disrupted by raids of DEA agents and arrests, reflecting the clash of two very different value systems. In spite of the controversies surrounding him, our personal connection was strong enough that my fiancée and I chose to invite him to our wedding in 1966. Timothy respectfully declined, but gifted us with a copy of his *Psychedelic Prayers*, his own adaptation of the first book of the Tao Tê Ching, attractively published on embossed paper. Earlier, with Richard Alpert and Ralph Metzner, he had published *The Psychedelic Experience: A Manual Based on the Tibetan Book of the Dead*, a guidebook for navigating within alternative states of awareness that still remains helpful for people preparing for psychedelic sessions.

Two images stand out for me in my memories of the psychedelic community at Millbrook. One is a once-magnificent but now defunct fountain in front of the mansion, overgrown with weeds, that no one seemed motivated to repair. The other was a deserted bowling alley, artistically designed as a long, separate building with a high ceiling, located in a quiet woodland setting, which was also neglected and abandoned. When I saw it, I immediately imagined how it could be transformed into a very distinctive meditation hall. There was a small square building designated for meditation near the mansion with pillows on the floor, but, like the rest of the estate, it was dusty and poorly maintained. As a whole, I felt as though Millbrook was a secular ashram or monastery with hardly any structure or discipline. It is not surprising that it proved unable to sustain itself.

The image of a classic Tibetan mandala comes to mind, a symmetrical design made up of concentric squares and circles, one within the other, with gates on each of the four sides of the squares, leading to a central point of meditative focus. Insofar as such mandalas depict the healthy, centered psyche, there is a balance between squares and circles. Squares, rectangular lines, and right angles in art therapy tend to be interpreted as manifestations of the masculine or active pole of our minds: cognition, reason, structure, decisions, commitment, assertive behavior. Circular or curved forms, in contrast, are understood to reflect the feminine or passive pole: receptivity, trust, patience, openness, gentleness. It has always been fascinating to me to observe how people struggling with alcoholism tend to produce artwork dominated by curved, paisley-type lines, whereas those struggling with obsessive-compulsive tendencies tend to rely almost exclusively on rigid, straight lines. From my perspective, the community at Millbrook urgently needed a wise and stern abbot and the position appeared vacant. Paisley forms dominated there, at least when I happened to visit.

It is easy for present psychedelic researchers to complain about Timothy Leary and make him a scapegoat for the three decades of lost research progress from which we are just recovering. In all fairness, however, it should be acknowledged that, with his colleagues, he did publish some significant research studies and attempted to communicate cogently with academic colleagues before he abandoned traditional science in favor of seeking attention through a sensationalistic press. For example, he published a report in the *Journal of Nervous and Mental Disease* that included statistical analyses of the responses of

175 volunteers to whom he had administered questionnaires following their psilocybin experiences. He also spearheaded a creative pilot study that explored the use of psilocybin in the rehabilitation of thirty-two inmates from the Concord State Prison, a maximum-security facility for young offenders. Earlier in his career, he had published a respected book, *The Interpersonal Diagnosis of Personality*. Also, some compassion is in order for a single troubled human being who had struggled with alcohol abuse in the past and who found himself as a single parent of two young children after the suicide of his first wife. He was a colorful and tragic human being, but only one person among many dedicated clinicians and researchers in the early days of psychedelic studies.

It is thought provoking to reflect on how differently his two primary associates responded to their psychedelic experiences. Richard Alpert went to India, changed his name to Ram Dass, became established as a respected meditation teacher, and helped to create the Hanuman Foundation and the Seva Foundation, which have reached out to serve prisoners, the terminally ill, and the homeless. Ralph Metzner continues to have a productive career, has brought the Green Earth Foundation into being, and has called attention to nature, to the care of our planet, and to the respectful, spiritual use of ayahuasca.

INTEGRATING RELIGIOUS EXPERIENCES
INTO RELIGIOUS LIVES

Huston Smith, as noted earlier, was among the first to articulate a distinction between religious experiences and religious lives, having observed that the first does not automatically guarantee the latter. This is true not only of mystical experiences, whether facilitated by entheogens or by other technologies or seeming to occur naturally, but also of conversion, prayer, and meditative experiences of many varieties. Perhaps the principle extends beyond experiences we call religious to any profound and intense episodes or adventures in life—other peak or nadir experiences and even those experiences we label as traumatic.

To some extent some people seem to have a choice between "sealing off" the emotions and insights from experiences that break through the limits of routine, everyday reality or choosing to expend effort to work toward their integration. Some experiences bring with them a transformed sense of self and a strong impetus toward changed behavior in the world; others seem to "sit there" as intriguing memories that could remain isolated from daily routines. I recall a successful business leader who had a spontaneous mystical experience while lying on my office couch that met all the criteria in the definition of mystical consciousness. When he subsequently sat up on the couch, he said, "That was nice. What is it good for?" He had only glimpsed *samadhi*, the spiritual goal of life for many in Eastern religions.

There are no indications that St. Paul required a second vision of the risen Christ after his experience on the Road to Damascus; he experienced a shift in his view of the world and set off on a mission. Yet even he may well have valued the companionship and support of others as he sought to help establish and stabilize the fledgling congregations of early Christianity. Many of the research volunteers who have encountered profoundly spiritual experiences during the action of psilocybin at Johns Hopkins, all well-functioning people to begin with, have subsequently addressed issues of career or human relationships and reconfigured parts of their lives as they have progressed in the integration of their newfound knowledge. As examples, one person resigned from a job that entailed contributing to the design of military weaponry and a few years later was ordained as a Zen monk; another chose to join the Peace Corps and move to Africa.

What we call integration seems to entail a repetitive, intentional movement within awareness between memories from alternative states of consciousness and the demands and opportunities of everyday existence, including former habits of thought or action that may feel out of sync with the new knowledge or self-concept. For instance, the person who has suffered from alcoholism and who during the action of an entheogen has experienced a sense of unconditional love and acceptance cannot return to the former feelings of low self-worth and wallow in them without feeling a disconnect and a need for integration. He or she may well feel humility, but it arises not out of a sense of worthlessness but rather out of awe and reverence.

The gradual process of integrating religious experiences is often assisted by participation in supportive communities. It is here that one may value belonging to a church, temple, synagogue, mosque, or group of some kind where one can speak of one's insights, hear about those of others, and unite in practical applications that may effect social and cultural change. Along with such social involvement, many may find instruction in and the committed practice of meditative disciplines significantly helpful. Within community life, one may also learn a language with which to express the insights that have occurred and may find it easier to adjust to changing patterns of attitudes and behavior. Those who have struggled with addictions may especially value participation in Alcoholic, Narcotic, or Overeaters Anonymous fellowships. If more churches, synagogues, temples, mosques, and sanghas offered support and study groups for those who had experienced profound alternate states of consciousness, whether engendered by entheogen use or occurring in other ways, the number of people responding could be surprising.

For some, the process of integration may be aided by a period of counseling, psychotherapy, or spiritual direction. When this occurs, it need not be assumed that one was damaged by a psychedelic experience and thus requires treatment or spiritual support to return to a prior baseline condition. Rather, especially when people uncover traumatic memories, often of physical, verbal, or sexual abuse, that have been sealed away within their minds, interaction with a skilled therapist may prove very helpful in assimilating those memories into the overall functioning of the mind, thereby decreasing chronic anxiety and depression and facilitating the establishment of a more mature, better-integrated identity. Such treatment or disciplined interpersonal interaction may prove to be hard work, but the rewards can be significantly meaningful.

12

Reflections on Death

There was a time in Western societies, not very long ago, when one didn't talk about sex in polite company. Sexual fantasies and behavior, either interpersonal or personal, tended to be very private and often guilt-ridden. Psychiatrists frequently encountered people in whom sexual anxieties had become manifested as conversion symptoms, such as impotence and frigidity, sometimes with actual paralysis. Now in most circles men and women can speak of sexuality with reasonable openness and sensitivity without being viewed as depraved or vulgar. Women can view being orgasmic and desiring sexual interaction as indicators of good health. In some circles even people committed to celibacy can experience occasional orgasms with gratitude rather than feelings of failure and guilt. Increasingly some people can now even honestly own both heterosexual and homosexual fantasies without undue self-doubt, regardless of their choice of adult sexual identity.

While sex may be seen as "coming out of the closet," the closet door still tends to be tightly closed for many of us when it comes to death. The topic still often remains taboo, surrounded by vague fears and muddled thoughts. Some of us still view death as an unpleasant event that sometimes happens to other people. Many prefer to not even begin to come to terms with the awareness that everyone who has ever lived on this planet has eventually died and there is a very high probability that each of us will also die someday.

What then, we may ask, is death really? Observed from without, we picture a human body that ceases to function. The heart slows and stops beating. The breathing ceases. The skin grows cold. Rigor mortis sets in. Soon the faint sweet scent of decomposition begins as the walls of cells begin to collapse. The person with whom we could once interact with speech and gestures is gone, never to return. Grief intensifies.

If the intuitive knowledge of mystics is taken seriously, what then might the experience we call death be like for the person who we declare "dead"? If consciousness is really indestructible, what adventures might await us? As one who has pondered this question with many different terminally ill people who have suddenly decided that the topic is of importance, I can report that there is a considerable range of expectations.

Some expect awareness to simply end, like "a lightbulb going out," and may even express some anxiety that this might not be the case. There are those who feel they've had enough of life and would rather not have more of it, eternal or otherwise, joyful or painful. They are weary and exhausted with constricted awareness and simply aren't interested in exciting new adventures. Others hope to move through different states of consciousness, realms of hell, purgatory, or heaven, or all three, perhaps to deal with judgment of how this lifetime has been lived, perhaps to reunite with beloved relatives and friends, ancestors and religious figures, who have lived before. Some hope for simple peace and heavenly bliss, at least for a while; others who take reincarnation seriously may imagine physical rebirth and "doing the diaper thing again."

The Bardo Thodol, the sacred text known as the Tibetan Book of the Dead, treats the changes of consciousness after the body stops functioning very much like a psychedelic experience. How one responds to the changes in consciousness, especially in terms of focused attention, acceptance, humility, trust, and courage, it is believed, may well influence "what happens next." In many Christian circles, it is believed that if one entrusts one's life to the archetypal Christ, or, more simply expressed, if one "gives one's heart to Jesus," one is indeed "saved" and all will ultimately be well.

The five-letter English word "death," like the three-letter word "God" is one of those sounds we emit in speech that can have significantly different meanings for different people. If consciousness is truly indestructible, death simply is a word for transition, or perhaps for "waking up" to a more vivid awareness of our spiritual nature. This was the point that the Russian novelist Leo Tolstoy sought to communicate in his short story *The Death of Ivan Ilyich*. He described Ivan's experience of the moment of his death as follows:

> "And death? Where is it?" He tried to find his former customary fear of death, and could not. "Where is death? What is it?" There was no fear, because there was no death. In the place of death was light! "Here is something like," he suddenly said aloud. "What joy." For him all this passed in a single instant, and the significance of this instant did not change. . . . "It is over! Death!" he said to himself. "It does not exist more."

What would civilization look like if most of us no longer feared death? What if "life" were understood to include states of consciousness expressed both in the context of normally functioning physical organisms and in energetic fields of awareness quite invisible to ordinary sensory perception? What if the everyday consciousness of most people was sufficiently enlightened or awake to include awareness of both the temporal and the eternal dimensions of a greater reality? This awakened awareness is of course a goal of many people dedicated to meditative disciplines, both Western and Eastern.

It sometimes seems as though we tend to be "afraid of not fearing death," anxious that, if death is not intrinsically evil and to be avoided whenever possible, we might all suddenly become more prone to suicide or homicide. Some might tend to magnify these fears by recalling images of tragedies of the past, such as the multiple deaths at the compound in Guyana led by Jim Jones, the harms inflicted by suicide bombers, or the carnage in battlefields throughout history.

Yet the evidence from psychedelic research provides little support for such fears. People who lose their fear of death typically appear to live more fully, to respect their own lives and the evolving lives of others, and to treasure the time that remains in interaction with family and friends. Some cancer patients may choose to forgo final experimental procedures that have little probability of offering extended duration of qualitative life. But as long as pain can be managed and meaningful communication is possible, which is usually possible with modern medical care, they appear eager to continue to do whatever is required to keep their bodies functioning. From this perspective it would appear that the reason to keep our bodies functioning for as long as meaningful life is possible is not to avoid the horror of death, but rather to fulfill our destinies as completely as possible. For some, that may entail completing creative work, cleaning up the messes we have made, preparing those we love to continue their lives without us, or simply savoring every moment that is given to us in the world of time.

A PERSONAL ENCOUNTER WITH DEATH

After debating within myself how self-disclosing to be in this book, not wanting it to be self-indulgent or excessively autobiographical, I have decided to illustrate this discussion by describing the death of Ilse, my wife for twenty years. The mother of my two sons, Ilse was a psychiatric nurse from Germany who often worked with me in psychedelic research. Together we had interacted with many cancer patients, their spouses, and their children in the context of providing brief counseling assisted by one or two sessions of alternative states of consciousness facilitated by LSD. Ilse herself had received LSD and had experienced exquisitely beautiful and meaningful states of consciousness as part of her training when we first moved to Baltimore to pursue research at the Spring Grove Hospital Center. In those days, on-the-job training for new personnel who would be involved in clinical research with psychedelic substances always included one or two personal experiences with LSD. Ilse had also earned a diploma from three years of study at a Baptist theological seminary in Zurich called Rüschlikon and had pursued graduate studies in the psychology of religion in the United States at the Andover-Newton Theological School in Newton Centre, Massachusetts.

Thus, when she was diagnosed with breast cancer at age forty, we looked at each other in shocked bewilderment, but then affirmed that, if any couple was prepared to cope with this situation, we must be. During the next decade she lived fully and courageously as various surgeries, courses of radiation, chemotherapeutic regimens, and even a trip to Mexico to obtain an experimental substance we called "black goop" came and went. Finally, however, we reached that point where the image of her skeleton during the bone scan lit up with multiple metastases and we could feel with our fingertips the hard nodes of cancer advancing in her clavicles. We knew it was time to prepare our sons, then eleven and thirteen, for her approaching death and did so together as sensitively as we could.

A few weeks later, after the accumulating fluid in her pleural cavity had been drained for a second time, we knew that death was imminent. She was still ambulatory, did not require narcotic pain medications, and was fully present with us in our home. We had opted not to accept a final highly experimental offer of chemotherapy that might well have provided slightly more quantity of life at the expense of quality.

She walked upstairs for the last time and, lying in bed beside each son, one at a time, reaffirmed all those things a son needs to hear from his mother. One son tape-recorded his final conversation, including, "I wish you didn't have to die, Mommy," evoking the response, "I wish I didn't either, but we have to accept life as it is." I then tucked our boys into their beds and lay beside her as the moment of death approached. Her final words were "Herr, Herr, Herr" (Lord, Lord, Lord) and she then entered into progressively deepening coma and the cessation of her bodily functions. Those final words suggested that, in spite of her advanced knowledge of comparative religions and transcendental states of mind, the simple faith of her Christian childhood effectively manifested itself at the moment of death. Steve Jobs, in a contrasting variation of words on the threshold of death, was reported by his sister to have uttered, "Oh wow, Oh wow, Oh wow."

Though inevitably painful–griefwork is never fun–Ilse's death occurred with negligible depression and anxiety, and with close communication with those she loved. She did not understand why it needed to occur at age fifty while our sons were still young and she still had many plans for this lifetime. Yet, possessing the knowledge from the mystical experiences in which she had participated, she lived with an intuitive conviction that there is a bigger framework of understanding where all makes sense and all is well.

This is one of many examples of a "good death," at least one approached with the openness, honesty, and courage that seem to promote fullness of living, prior to death for the terminally ill person and after death for the friends and family members who survive. There are many people who have never had mystical experiences or opportunities to receive entheogens who, on the basis of their belief systems and interpersonal connections alone, manifest a similar sense of peaceful integration on their deathbeds. However, there are also many who approach the end of their lives with notable anxiety, deep depression, and withdrawal from meaningful interaction with life companions. For the former, the vivid memory of mystical consciousness could well further enhance their sense of well-being on the threshold of death; for the latter, it might open up the possibility of finding meaning and dramatically decreasing emotional and physical distress.

GRIEFWORK

As those who have grieved or are currently grieving know well, grief is indeed work. And on the level of human biology in the world of time, grief seems to need to run its course no matter how spiritually elevated one's belief system concerning death may be. As one who has taught college courses in death and dying, I discovered new, experiential knowledge about the process and pain of grieving following Ilse's death, especially in terms of the physical, somatic manifestations. Grief does appear to be a healing process and, just as childbirth is not without pain, the process of reorienting oneself in the world after the loss of a beloved person does seem to progress in meaningful patterns, especially when one is able to trust one's own emotions and allow their expression.

The confrontation of unresolved grief and its expression and resolution is a common occurrence during the action of psychedelic substances. Not infrequently, the losses being grieved occurred decades earlier at a time when, whether due to emotional ambivalence, a lack of social support, or other factors, people chose to "be strong," deny their feelings, "put the death behind them," and rapidly move ahead with life. It appears that those repressed feelings patiently await opportunities for resolution, and while waiting may well engender muscular tensions, tendencies toward depression and anxiety, and psychosomatic distress symptoms for some people. Claims of increased freedom and relaxation are often made following the catharsis of grief, not only for those who have lost loved ones in the past, but also prospectively for terminally ill people who also need to grieve the imminent loss of all they have known in life. The unexpected encounter with repressed grief is one common theme in many psychedelic experiences that become labeled as "bad trips."

CHANGING ATTITUDES TOWARD DEATH

Now, what if more of us were to experience our own deaths and the deaths of those we love in ways characterized by honesty, openness, and trust? The implications of such a change in the manner our culture tends to cope with death would be profound in terms of preventive medicine. Many forms of psychological distress either originate in or are exacerbated by unresolved conflicts in interpersonal relationships– words of acceptance and forgiveness that were never spoken. Old hurts and resentments, expressed in anxieties, depressive tendencies, rigid judgments, and tense muscles, often have a way of enduring long after the people who perpetuated them have died.

Many doctors and nurses in recent years appear to have become more comfortable and skilled in honestly discussing issues of diagnosis and prognosis with those who are seriously or terminally ill. This of course requires them to do some deep introspection themselves and to begin to come to terms with their own mortality. I recall an elderly African American cancer patient who learned her diagnosis and prognosis while seated in her hospital bathroom, overhearing her doctor as he spoke to a group of residents in the hallway outside the door of her room, before entering. The first issue she introduced as we began meeting together in preparation for a psychedelic session was, "Should I tell my doctor that I know? Can he take it?"

I often think of how the option of receiving psychedelic therapy could be integrated into the palliative care units of our hospitals and perhaps into our hospices. When I was pursuing my doctoral research, a study with DPT in promoting the well-being of cancer patients in close proximity of their deaths, the term "hospice" referred to an innovative experiment being conducted by Dr. Cicely Saunders at a single site she founded for caring for terminally ill people called St. Christopher's in London. Now, hospices have become accepted social institutions with coverage provided by Medicare and other insurance companies. The National Hospice and Palliative Care Organization (NHPCO) reported approximately thirty-four hundred Medicare-certified hospice providers in the United States in 2012.

Aldous Huxley, on the final day of his life, when critically ill with laryngeal cancer, wrote a request to his wife, Laura, stating, "Try LSD, 100 gamma, intramuscular." As described in Laura's memoir, *This Timeless Moment*, she complied with this final request and administered the LSD to him. When the response appeared minimal, she gave Aldous an additional 100 mcg a couple hours later, just before his actual death. Though this sacramental act may have been personally meaningful to Aldous, who had written in his novel *Island* about the "moksha medicine" administered at critical life junctures, and perhaps to Laura as well, this final gesture has always struck me as akin to sprinkling water on someone just before he or she dives into the ocean. It makes much more sense to me to integrate a treatment intervention with psychedelics into palliative care (defined as a prognosis of at least six months) or even to offer it as an option to people when cancer or another potentially life-threatening disease is first diagnosed. The longer the time period when one may be more acutely conscious of a larger reality and interact meaningfully with significant others while experiencing decreased anxiety, depression, and pain, the better.

Attitudes toward death are changing. An example is Agrace Hospice and Palliative Care in Madison, Wisconsin, where many rooms open to private courtyards so, if one so desires, one can choose to die under the open sky instead of in a hospital room. There, those who have cared for a person may accompany the corpse, head uncovered, in a procession down the hallway to a hearse at the front entrance of the facility instead of discretely sending it down an elevator in a closed body bag, it is hoped when no one is watching, to the typical rear loading dock. When death is more fully accepted, whether in hospices or in private homes, there are many more opportunities for genuine communication and even for music and laughter. After all, what if someone is simply "waking up"? The Buddha, as many know, is the "one who woke up" and perhaps there is a potential Buddha within us all.

A memory arises from visiting Varanasi, the holiest of Indian cities for Hindu people. There I stood beside the Manikarnika Ghat, one of the "burning ghats" where cremations almost constantly proceed on steps that descend into the sacred river Ganges. Hindus traditionally believe that, if one dies in Varanasi (also known as Benares or Kashi), one goes straight to heaven. I watched male relatives sitting in a straight line watching a corpse burn. It had been immersed in the Ganges, carefully prepared with ghee and sandalwood, decorated with flowers, and wrapped in cloth of symbolic significance. It then had been placed on a stack of branches and logs, carefully calculated to provide the intensity and length of heat required to complete the cremation. Often the oldest son, wearing the traditional white Dhoti, ignites a torch at the nearby temple where the eternal flame always burns and carries it to the funeral pyre. After walking around it five times clockwise (symbolizing the elements, earth, air, fire, water, and ether), he ignites the pyre. Sometimes at the appropriate time, he may even take a bamboo pole and crush the skull to ensure that the flames consume the brain.

While this ritual was occurring, which most Westerners would view as incredibly somber, if not grotesque, young teenage boys were running and laughing, joyfully playing cricket in full view of the cremation in the very next ghat, with no barrier between. The acceptance of death as an integral part of life appeared so well established that, if a cricket ball had landed in the cremation pyre, I doubt that anyone would have been unduly upset. After about three or four hours of burning, the ashes and remaining bone fragments are poured into the Ganges and the relatives walk away, traditionally without looking back. Death is part of life and in Varanasi it is common to see grandfather's body, wrapped in a blanket and strapped to the top of a station wagon, moving through the narrow streets en route to cremation. It is mind-boggling for me to compare this with some of our Western funerary procedures. How often have I stood beside a corpse laid out in an expensive casket in an American funeral home with a rose-colored lamp focused on the face to help it look lifelike while people standing beside me awkwardly comment about "how good he looks." Do we still tend to suffer from denial of death?

In interactions with terminally ill people and their families, I consider it important to respect whatever belief systems or lack thereof one encounters. Insofar as is possible, if one desires to be helpful, the goal is to meet people where they are and to speak in ways that may be comprehensible and supportive. If someone expects nothing after death, it is possible to discuss what that expectation may feel like, just as one may discuss anticipation of hellish or heavenly states of mind or of encountering one's ancestors. As in any good human interaction, honest, nonjudgmental communication tends to relieve anxiety and facilitate the resolution of guilt and anger, promoting feelings of acceptance, forgiveness, and sometimes even a touch of playfulness. It is reasonable to expect that whatever is or is not going to happen after death will probably occur no matter what our beliefs or expectations may be. What matters is not the acceptance of ideas, but the acceptance of love, perhaps both human and divine.

The counseling process, akin to other genuine interpersonal interactions, also tends to relax muscular tensions that sometimes may have exacerbated physical pain. The meaning of pain often shifts during psychedelic therapy from a threatening herald of death in the central focus of awareness to a sensation somewhere in the periphery of one's field of consciousness. Following effective therapy, relationships have become central–with oneself, with others, and with whatever one considers sacred. Repeatedly I have heard, "The pain is still there, but it doesn't bother me like before."

From the perspective of mystical consciousness, the universe is so awesomely vast that there is room for unlimited variations of immortal life. In the West, we tend to forget that many people in the East take reincarnation for granted with the same lack of discernment that we manifest in usually dismissing it as a realistic option. When it comes to immortality, for whatever it may be worth, I do not feel any need for a "one size fits all" approach. Perhaps some of us do reincarnate some times. Ian Stevenson, a psychiatrist at the University of Virginia, documented some rather convincing case histories for those who are open to the possibility. He interviewed people who claimed to remember a prior lifetime and then pursued detailed detective work to try to confirm the information provided.

Perhaps even those who expect nothing after death might get to experience that until it becomes too boring, or until it becomes recognized as the Buddhist "nothingness that contains all reality." Some of us, whether we expect it or not, may well encounter loved ones and ancestors and archetypal manifestations within consciousness such as angels and demons. The literature on near-death experiences, reports of those who have entered into the physical processes of death and have been resuscitated, contains many intriguing stories to ponder that are often very similar to psychedelic experiences, complete with reports of moving through tunnels, encountering visionary beings, and being drawn toward sacred realms of light. However, regardless of the content that may occur after death, I can report the repeated observation that, with trust, openness, and interpersonal grounding, anxiety often becomes displaced by simple, honest curiosity and a capacity to serenely accept life as it is.

PART IV

*Present and Future Applications
of Entheogens*

13

Psychedelic Frontiers in Medicine

THE USE OF ENTHEOGENS IN PSYCHOTHERAPY

There is an abundance of published studies that strongly suggest that the use of psychedelic substances may be of significant value in the treatment of numerous mental health conditions. In the hands of skilled therapists, who can establish solid rapport and who understand the art of navigating within the human mind, psychedelics may be understood as tools that can intensify, deepen, and significantly accelerate the healing processes of psychotherapy. Claims are frequently made that some single psychedelic experiences are equivalent to several years of regular appointments for psychotherapeutic treatment. It would be easy to dismiss such words as irresponsible exaggeration and enthusiasm, were not some of them spoken by people who are themselves professional therapists and have personally pursued years of more conventional treatment.

The time is ripe to competently design and implement projects of research focused on the inclusion of psychedelics in the treatment of people who are experiencing particular forms of distress. From all we have learned, it seems established that such treatment must be carried out in the context of healthy human relationships. Simply prescribing an entheogen as a purely chemotherapeutic medication appears unlikely to be helpful for very many people. At the time of writing, new studies with psychedelics are focusing on the treatment of addictions to alcohol, heroin, cocaine, and nicotine, states of anxiety and depression, and, in one study, high-functioning people suffering from autism and Asperger's Syndrome. As described elsewhere, there are many options for investigating the use of psychedelic substances in psychotherapy, in the past labeled as psycholytic, psychedelic, and psychodelytic and more recently integrated with cognitive-behavioral approaches to treatment and procedures for enhancing motivation. Different psychoactive substances may be investigated in varying doses, in different treatment milieus, varying the frequency and dosage of entheogen administration, the time spent in individual and group process, coordination with supplemental therapeutic procedures, the overall duration of treatment, and opportunities for follow-up care or periodic retreatment.

For example, initial results from a recent project at Johns Hopkins directed by Matthew Johnson and Albert Garcia-Romeu that employed psilocybin and cognitive-behavioral techniques in the treatment of nicotine addiction have been very promising. A pilot study of fifteen mentally and physically healthy people who had repeatedly failed attempts to overcome their nicotine addictions, smoking an average of nineteen cigarettes per day for an average of thirty-one years, found an abstinence rate of 80 percent six months after a brief treatment intervention that included a maximum of three psilocybin sessions. This research is continuing with a larger controlled study and, if these results hold up, the public health implications are staggering. According to the Centers for Disease Control and Prevention (CDC), tobacco is considered the leading preventable cause of death, credited with causing five million deaths per year worldwide, including 480,000 annually in the United States alone. Here is a frontier of great potential significance for improving human health that is wide open to medically trained personnel who would like to better understand the factors that are proving effective and perhaps even to improve on them.

Similarly, Michael Bogenschutz, resurrecting promising prior research that employed LSD or DPT in the treatment of people suffering from alcoholism, has completed a pilot study with ten volunteers at the University of New Mexico who received psilocybin in the context of interpersonal support and Motivational Enhancement Therapy. He has found that intense, often mystical experiences during the action of psilocybin strongly predicted decreased alcohol consumption and craving one week after psilocybin administration, gains that were largely maintained when patients were interviewed and tested six months after treatment. As with volunteers struggling with nicotine addiction, no significant treatment-related adverse events were observed. A larger controlled study investigating the contribution psilocybin may make in the treatment of alcoholism currently is underway at New York University at a rapidly expanding center for the treatment of addictions spearheaded by Stephen Ross and his colleagues.

Research projects employing psychotherapy assisted by psychedelic drugs with cancer patients suffering from depression, anxiety, interpersonal isolation, and pain, both in the 1960s and early 1970s and since such research has resumed, have reported significantly reduced psychological and physical distress in many of the participants. This hopeful finding tends to be understood not as a pharmacological response, akin to regularly taking an antidepressant or tranquillizing medication, but rather as the enduring response to one, or at most three, journeys within consciousness and the vivid memories of those experiences. It is worthy of note that, although most current research projects with normal volunteers disqualify applicants with histories of serious depressive episodes, current researchers regularly receive unsolicited testimonials by people who claim that a single entheogenic experience saved them from deep depression and serious suicidal ideation. At the present time, researchers at the Imperial College of London are beginning to probe the promise of psychedelics in treating depression, examining biochemical and neuroimaging parameters as well as clinical data. There are many opportunities to replicate or further explore their findings.

A potentially important area of research, as yet almost untouched, is the use of entheogens in the treatment of persons with sociopathic personality disorders. These people, whether due to genetic inclinations, childhood trauma and neglect, or inadequate opportunities and structure during their formative years, often seem to find it difficult to experience meaningful connections with others and thus to experience concomitant feelings of responsibility, genuine caring, guilt, and remorse. As their lives progress, many of them get arrested for violating the moral or legal standards of our society and then spend years being minimally productive while they occupy prison cells. In 2014, a criminal justice research and advocacy group called the Prison Policy Initiative published a report estimating that 2.4 million people are chronically imprisoned in the United States, not counting those who are briefly locked up and released. This situation, unparalleled in the world, requires and nourishes a massive industry of prison construction, staffing, and maintenance, as well as courts and legal personnel. For those of us who freely walk the streets, "out of sight, out of mind" applies. Whenever I have entered a prison to visit a person, I have been almost rudely shocked out of my complacency. The world of caged people, of barren walls often painted pink, of high decibels of noise, of disrespect, intimidation, fear, and despair can clearly qualify as an example of hell on earth.

There are many who share my belief that a society that really cared about all its citizens could creatively address this problem. After all, we've demonstrated that we can put men on the moon if we decide it is a national priority. Among the interventions that merit serious funding and exploration is psychotherapy assisted by the use of psychedelic substances. Why give drugs to convicts? Simply expressed, because in the context of healthy relationships with a skilled treatment staff, sufficient trust gradually could well be developed to make positive psychodynamic and mystical experiences possible. Traumatized and neglected people could conceivably experience healing, bonding, and "reparenting." When mystical consciousness occurs and is vividly remembered, there is finally knowledge of love and belonging to the family of humanity that might well make possible changes in self-concept, forgiveness of self and others, and the construction of a code of personal ethics. The new knowledge would require integration and reinforcement in the context of group therapy, constructive employment, and decent housing.

One study in the scientific literature in which psilocybin was administered to thirty-four inmates in the Concord Prison in Massachusetts between 1961 and 1963 by Timothy Leary, Ralph Metzner, and their colleagues at Harvard University showed promise but, perhaps due to the experimental design and the lack of adequately supportive after-care, did not demonstrate enduring results in terms of recidivism. Around the same time, a study by B. Tenenbaum of the treatment of ten criminal sex offenders incarcerated in the Atascadero State Hospital in California and a study by G. W. Arendsen-Hein, who gave a series of LSD sessions to twenty-one chronic criminal offenders in the Netherlands, were published, both of which indicated promising results. No psychedelic substance is a "magic bullet" that will permanently cure any condition, akin to taking an aspirin tablet to dispel a common headache. However, the wise use of these substances may well nurture sufficient personal and spiritual growth to significantly change attitudes and behavior, especially when combined with well-funded supportive services.

In evaluating many different projects that have employed psychedelics in medical treatment, there appears to have been a tendency to conclude that, if enduring miracles fail to easily occur, the substances have no value at all. A more sober approach is clearly appropriate and in order. Also, to reiterate once again, it is not the simple administration of the psychedelic substance that promotes healing and facilitates personal and spiritual maturation; it is the discrete states of consciousness that are skillfully facilitated and experienced during the period of entheogen action and their subsequent memory and integration that constitute the effective healing principles.

ADVANCES IN UNDERSTANDING HEALING PROCESSES

Some recent developments in psychoanalytic theory and treatment may reasonably be focused to accommodate the responsible use of entheogens. Wilfred Bion, a British psychoanalyst who lived from 1897 until 1979, for example, often quoted the phrase "the deep and formless infinite" from John Milton's *Paradise Lost*, and referred to Ultimate Reality or God with his term "O." Though usually considered a "secular mystic," he acknowledged sacredness and mystery within human consciousness without devaluing it.

Carl Jung, as recently discussed in a scholarly and insightful book by Scott Hill, similarly had deep respect for what he called "the transcendent function" and called attention to the collective unconscious, the organized realm of archetypes discovered in human consciousness that appears intrinsic to our being, quite independent of the complexes we develop in our early childhoods. Though Bion and Jung have died and cannot participate in current psychedelic research, the opportunity is now becoming available for similar psychoanalytic theorists and clinicians to further explore the depths of consciousness and processes of healing with the assistance of entheogens. As in the study of mystical literature, one can look beyond the analysis of the writings of seminal psychoanalytic theorists and empirically explore the depths of the mind. The image of the seer pointing at the moon is germane: instead of studying the seer's finger, true disciples could look in the direction that the seer was pointing, make their own discoveries, consult with colleagues, design research projects of their own, and formulate refreshingly new hypotheses and conclusions.

When one takes seriously the perspective from the pinnacle of mystical consciousness, accepting the more fundamental reality of the eternal dimension of mind, the manner in which we understand the role of the therapist (psychiatrist, psychologist, social worker, psychiatric nurse, pastoral counselor, or shaman) in the healing process may shift. If the ultimate healing force is the energy we call love that flows into time from the sacred dimensions of consciousness, the healer becomes the conduit or facilitator. Instead of performing ingenious procedures and techniques, however clever and supported by complex theoretical constructs they may be, the healer's primary task may be understood as getting his or her ego out of the way and becoming fully present, as if focusing a beam of light that comes from beyond. Clark Martin, a psychologist who has publicly discussed his prior personal history of anxiety associated with cancer, has recently written that, on the basis of his experiences as a research volunteer at Johns Hopkins several years ago, he now considers the "presence" of the therapist even more fundamentally important than "empathy" in effective mental health treatment, in part because it is not dependent on language. One manifestation of this theoretical adjustment has been his teaching of mindfulness in conjunction with his clinical services.

In a particular MDA experience, this healing process was vividly symbolized by light penetrating through a stained-glass window, providing clarity, warmth, and unconditional acceptance. If the window symbolizes the therapist, the uniqueness of the healer's personal life may well constitute the pigments that refract and color the energies of the eternal light. One may appreciate the art of the unique therapist; however, it may well be that the being of the therapist matters more than the words the therapist speaks, the actions offered, or the concepts employed to theoretically articulate what is occurring. Within this metaphor, the ideal, fully enlightened therapist is "transparent to transcendence"; in reality therapists manifest different degrees of translucency on different days and hope not to become so preoccupied with their personal issues and agendas that they become experienced as opaque.

If the word "God" is used to describe this ultimate love in the core of being, then it makes sense to say that, in the healing process, God works through imperfect human beings, often called wounded healers, and "does everything that matters." It also becomes important to acknowledge that this love is also manifested in and through the client, directed toward the therapist as well, where it may be received and acknowledged appropriately. Although the psychoanalytic concepts of transference and countertransference may capture stages and distortions in this process, it also becomes of importance to acknowledge the genuineness of "the real relationship" that may be emerging, as has been emphasized by the existential-humanistic psychologist James Bugental. This applies not only to psychotherapy, but also to other genuinely helpful forms of personal interaction, whether called spiritual direction, life coaching, or solidly vital human relationships.

With the renewed interest in psychedelic substances and the ways indigenous healers or shamans have employed them, there is the potential to learn more than how the molecules in certain plant substances may be synthesized in the medicines of the future. Instead of arrogantly viewing shamans as primitive "witch doctors" who have been deprived of the brilliant knowledge of Western allopathic medicine, it is becoming increasingly apparent that some shamans indeed possess valuable knowledge to share with us, not only concerning exotic herbs and concoctions, but also about techniques of navigating within consciousness and the spiritual interconnectedness of us all. The sharing of knowledge and worldviews in the respectful interaction of professional healers, whether in Brazil, Tibet, Gabon, the United States, or elsewhere, is likely to prove to be a win-win situation for all.

INVESTIGATING CORRELATIONS BETWEEN
BRAIN ACTIVITY AND CONSCIOUSNESS

Psychedelic substances appear to have significant promise as tools in the rapidly expanding field of cognitive neuroscience. Studies are being conducted in which experienced "psychonauts" who are familiar with a variety of alternate states of consciousness and who have mastered basic skills of navigating in these inner worlds agree to participate in research projects in which they lie in Positron Emission Tomography (PET) scanners or noisy Functional Magnetic Resonance Imaging (fMRI) machines, allowing their brain activity to be scanned, physiological parameters to be monitored, and samples of bodily fluids to be collected. Even when these highly experienced explorers of human consciousness agree to serve as volunteer subjects in such experiments, care is required to ensure an interpersonally comfortable relationship with the investigators and a warm and safe research environment.

Scientists can thus attempt to study the correlations between blood flow in specific areas of their volunteers' brains (presumed to indicate the intensity of activity), chemical changes in their blood samples, and similar data with the inner states of consciousness reported and behavioral responses to different stimuli. Such studies are still in relatively early phases of development, with reports in professional journals sometimes referring to "the psychedelic state" rather than reflecting awareness of the incredible variety of psychedelic states, and sometimes appearing to unquestionably accept a belief that consciousness originates in brain activity, an assumption that many who personally have explored alternative states might consider inadequate and unnecessarily reductionistic.

Some of the most exciting recent studies have been taking place at the Imperial College in London by David Nutt and his colleagues, including Robin Carhart-Harris and David Erritzoe; at the University Hospital in Zurich under the direction of Franz Vollenweider; and at the Johns Hopkins School of Medicine in Baltimore by Roland Griffiths, Matthew Johnson, and Frederick Barrett. In a recent well-designed, placebo-controlled study by Rainer Kraehenmann and colleagues at the University of Zurich, for example, fMRI scans were obtained from twenty-five healthy young men, most of whom had no prior experience with entheogens, during the action of a low dose of psilocybin. They reported finding decreased reactivity in the amygdala, a key structure in serotonergic emotion-processing circuits, and suggested that additional research may support the effectiveness of psilocybin in the treatment of clinical depression.

It remains true, however, that, in spite of the exciting and important advances taking place in neuroscience, we still honestly do not know what we are. Philosophers and some scientists have been struggling with the mind-body problem for centuries, and no consensus has emerged yet. There is no question that our brains are involved in how we experience the complex cognitive, emotional, and volitional contents of our minds, perhaps akin to how a television set may affect and process the programs being received, but as stated earlier, that does not establish causation. As mentioned, the best answers to this conundrum we can come up with at this point in time may be formulated by theoretical physicists who are beginning to fathom the mysteries inherent in matter itself. Nonetheless, this research frontier in medicine may well lead to a more accurate understanding of brain functioning, may yield clues to help us develop new medications, and may uncover ways of more skillfully guiding us through many different states of awareness, both those we may desire and those we may wish to avoid or minimize such as severe states of depression or chronic obsessions and compulsions.

ENTHEOGENS IN THE TRAINING
OF MENTAL HEALTH PROFESSIONALS

Many training programs for mental health professionals require some amount of personal psychotherapy, not only to promote healthy practitioners, but also to enable them to learn something about how the human mind seems to work. This experiential learning could be significantly enhanced for many by some well-structured psychedelic sessions, once legal clearance for such educational ventures can be obtained. Just as reading about Paris, even in the French language, is no substitute for walking the streets of Paris, sitting in sidewalk cafes, interacting with its residents, and venturing into the Cathedral of Notre Dame and the exquisitely beautiful Gothic Chapel of Sainte Chapelle, so reading about the human mind is no substitute for deeply exploring it.

Besides gaining knowledge of the many different terrains within the mind, which is likely to increase the practitioner's empathy and effectiveness when working with future patients, sensitivity to the potency of factors such as trust, honesty, courage, and openness is likely to be enhanced. Experientially, one can come to understand how panic and paranoia are generated and how to effectively cope with those states of anxiety when they are encountered. One can also develop increased sensitivity for those times when unconditional positive regard clearly needs to be supplemented by the confident provision of firm structure and limits. Above all, however, experiential knowledge of visionary and mystical states might well endow practitioners with enhanced respect for the sacredness of the patients who seek their guidance, for the creative, integrative forces at work within us all, and for the miracle of life itself.

Eventually as programs are established to educate and certify practitioners in the science and art of using psychedelic substances in psychotherapy, some professionals will become qualified to judiciously employ entheogens in their clinics or private practices. Initial curricula and training programs are under development by the Multidisciplinary Association of Psychedelic Studies (MAPS), by the California Institute of Integral Studies (CIIS), and at New York University. Many mental health professionals were integrating psychedelic substances into their professional practices before the drugs were declared illegal, and there are healers and shamans in other cultures who have used them responsibly for hundreds of years and continue to do so.

REGARDING PURELY BIOCHEMICAL
EFFECTS OF ENTHEOGENS

Although the emphasis in this book is on the experiential dimensions occasioned by psychedelic substances, it should be noted that there appear to be purely biochemical factors that may also be of significance. As reported by Andrew Sewell, John Halpern, and Harrison Pope, for example, very low doses of psilocybin have been reported to offer relief for people who suffer from the excruciating pain of cluster headaches. An organization called Clusterbusters is pursuing this application. A new drug, called bromo-psilocybin, initially synthesized by Albert Hofmann, is being studied that has no noteworthy effects on consciousness, but reportedly helps many with headaches. Similar promise has been reported by Francisco Moreno and his colleagues in administering psilocybin in low dosage to people suffering from obsessive-compulsive disorder.

It may also be noted that there are people who have suggested that taking a very low, subthreshold dose of a psychedelic substance frequently, even on a daily basis, akin to a vitamin capsule, may enhance creativity and effective psychological functioning for some people. Though it has been suggested that this may be a purely biochemical effect, it could be that, if it works at all, it might work best for limited time periods in people who are already quite well integrated psychologically. I have no doubt that the biochemistry involved in what we consider good mental health and creativity is intricately complex, but the basic idea may not be as outrageous as it initially sounds. This is but one of many relatively simple and straightforward types of research projects awaiting careful investigation.

THE RELIGIOUS USE OF ENTHEOGENS
AND ADDICTIVE BEHAVIOR

In religious communities that value and employ entheogens as sacraments, there appears to be little alcohol or drug abuse. Further, it has been claimed that some members of such communities with histories of alcoholism or other addictions find the frequent administration of an entheogenic sacrament helpful in maintaining freedom from alcohol and drug dependence. For example, John Halpern and colleagues associated with the Harvard Medical School interviewed thirty-two American members of the Santo Daime religion, who had received ayahuasca in weekly church services. Twenty-four of the people interviewed had histories of dependence on alcohol or other drugs, twenty-two of whom were considered to be in full remission. Similar claims have been made by members of the Native American Church in the context of their sacramental use of peyote. These tantalizing claims clearly invite serious well-designed projects of research that are long overdue, but it is hoped will soon be implemented.

Testimonials by individual people who claim benefits from the use of entheogens that sound almost miraculous tend to be considered very skeptically in the scientific community, if at all. I was recently contacted by a man who claimed to have a history of two decades of addiction to methamphetamine and crack cocaine, who reported trying and failing inpatient drug rehabilitation programs on ten occasions, plus involvement in outpatient drug treatment centers and Alcoholics Anonymous support groups. He also acknowledged a twenty-year addiction to cigarette smoking, calling it "the most powerful addiction that I have ever experienced." He credits a mystical experience facilitated by psilocybin, along with cannabis use, in his gradual establishment of control over his addictions and now claims to have lived without methamphetamine, cocaine, or nicotine, or the tortuous cravings he once experienced, for almost six years. He considers psilocybin mushrooms integral, not only to his recovery but to his present religious life and would like to be able to legally take his sacrament of psilocybin in low dosage on a daily basis.

Another unsolicited testimonial has come from a man approaching age fifty who credits his use of ayahuasca approximately three times per month, integrated with his subsequent membership in the Santo Daime religion and his steady participation in Alcoholics Anonymous, with six years of successful recovery from multiple drug dependencies. He wrote as follows:

> I spent a good deal of my life as a chronic alcoholic of the hopeless variety. I also sustained a nearly uninterrupted, two-decades long dependence on opiates (mostly heroin and Oxycontin) and benzodiazepines. This diet did include a very ugly appetite for cocaine (mostly IV), but which was intermittent. I also used significant amounts of amphetamines in various forms over the years but to a lesser extent than the other substances just mentioned. After more than twenty years of bona fide addiction, my life was indeed a sad story of broken dreams. I had collapsed veins, missing teeth, many jail visits, treatment center stays, methadone clinic enrollments, Hepatitis C, no job, no girlfriend, and no life. By any standard, I was utterly hopeless. . . .

My Ceremonies [with ayahuasca] showed me, in a general way, my life in its totality. I was shown my gifts and my liabilities. I saw my blessings and my capacity for goodness but I was also shown my narcissism, my self-centeredness, my resentments, and my insecurities.

More importantly, though, I was given a clear vision of what I could become if I would only surrender my heart and my life to God and to His creation. The Fourth Step inventory and the Fifth Step confession of AA, often serious stumbling blocks for many, were made almost effortless for me through the ritual of ayahuasca. I became honest with myself and surrendered fully to the process, and without reservation. I proceeded rapidly on through the remaining Steps, and arrived at Step 12 with its cherished awakening in due course. In all reality, there is no "arriving"; the journey continues, one day at a time, for the rest of our lives. . . .

The awe-inspiring beauty of my visions coupled with the loving embrace of the Spirit of God (maternal, paternal, and fraternal aspects) dried my tears, soothed my pains, and allowed me to truly believe that all would be well. Words simply cannot capture the Love and acceptance I felt then, and which I continue to feel each day now.

Claims such as these invite the design of new pilot investigations to explore whether such stories reflect atypical responses or whether they constitute clues to new and perhaps exceptionally effective approaches to treatment that could significantly reduce the suffering of countless people who continue to struggle with severe and sometimes fatal addictions.

14

Psychedelic Frontiers
in Education

There is no question that there is knowledge to be had (that is, intuitive insights and understandings awaiting discovery) in many of the more intense and profound states of consciousness facilitated by psychedelic substances. These experiential realms of the human mind stand in sharp contrast to the mild states of varied sensory perception and often meaningless mental imagery typically encountered with low dosage and personal resistance. Knowledge may be gleaned on many levels, ranging from spiritual insights about the nature of one's own mind and its relationship to others and to the cosmos, to better understanding of the currents of the mind and how to navigate safely within them, to enhanced perception of the formative forces in one's childhood and how psychological tensions may find resolution, to specific insights relevant to many different academic disciplines.

Kenneth Tupper was among the first to articulate the potential value of entheogens in education. He has written about "existential intelligence" and has even suggested that we might consider a program for some adolescents called "Inward Bound" akin to "Outward Bound." In Tupper's words:

The development of the imaginative capacity to ponder one's place in the cosmos, of sensibilities of wonder and awe, and of mind-body awareness seems to receive comparatively short shrift in the present educational environment, where test scores and instrumental thinking still tend to preoccupy administrators, teachers and students. This is particularly true in the latter years of compulsory education, when many students in their teens seem to have lost the insatiable curiosity they had as children and to have instead become jaded and bored. The youthful exuberance for discovery, learning, and imagining is all too often displaced by a desire merely to unreflectively consume entertainment and material goods.

In this chapter, let us focus on the implications of entheogens for creativity and enhanced understanding in the humanities, as well as the natural and social sciences with a few relatively random vignettes.

PHILOSOPHY

Many readers are familiar with Plato's allegory of the cave. As presented in a dialogue in the *Republic* between Socrates and Plato's older brother, Glaucon, chained prisoners, immobile since childhood and unable to turn their heads, observe moving shadows on the wall they have always been facing within a cave. The shadows are caused by puppeteers waving replicas of objects such as trees, horses, and human figures (derived from the "real world") above their own heads with their backs to a fire inside the cave's mouth, their bodies hidden by a low wall. The perceptions of the prisoners constitute their reality; they know nothing of the puppeteers, the fire, life on the rolling hillside outside the mouth of the cave, or the brilliant sun. They've created words for each of the shadows and play games with one another predicting the order in which they may appear. Trees are obviously grey; green does not exist.

Finally, one prisoner is freed of his chains. Able to turn around and walk uphill, he discovers the fire and the puppeteers and, after initial reticence and confused bewilderment, gradually enters into the even greater reality beyond the mouth of the cave, adjusting first to the moon and then to the sun. He becomes a philosopher king. However, when he returns to the cave and tries to share his new knowledge with his fellow prisoners, he is ridiculed because his wild ideas go far beyond the conception of reality they have learned and with which they are comfortable. They conclude that the light has damaged his eyes and that he can no longer see properly and unanimously disapprove of anyone else leaving their cave. It now becomes the philosopher king's destiny to live among his companions within the cave and to try to gradually awaken them to a greater reality.

Understanding this allegory is obviously simple for any person who has experienced mystical consciousness. Plato died around 348 BCE; yet the insights he sought to express in his allegory are essentially the same as those that many who have experienced mystical forms of consciousness are striving to express today. Plato's world of forms, the realm of archetypes in the sunlight beyond the mouth of the cave that is considered more real than the perceptions of everyday existence, is a "place" that the mystic has indeed visited and remembers vividly. He has "been there," just as if he had made a trip to Machu Picchu or to the great pyramid of Giza. He has acquired indelible experiential learning.

For Platonic scholars, it becomes possible not only to understand Plato's ideas and writings more fully, but also to understand the probable origin of his view of the world. The knowledge that Plato belonged to the Eleusinian mystery religion wherein participants received a psychedelic brew called *kykeon* makes perfect sense, though it is conceivable that Plato could also have been a natural mystic whose innate biochemistry was sufficient to occasion mystical experiences without facilitation by entheogens. Today, however, with the assistance of psychedelic substances, it has become possible for scholars not only to study Plato's writings in the dark carrels of libraries, even in the original Greek, but also to visit the states of consciousness that inspired Plato's writings and confirm for themselves their nature and validity. Especially if Alfred North Whitehead was right in his assessment that most of Western philosophy since Plato has been "footnotes to Plato," this knowledge could be viewed as invaluable to any serious student of the discipline. What if universities offered an experiential seminar, perhaps called Philosophy 599, in which qualified students could legally receive a psychedelic substance in a context that offered skilled preparation and provided for maximum safety? Probably not all students in the seminar would experience the full mystical consciousness described by Plato in their first sessions. Some would find alternative states of thought and perception that would help them understand the perspectives of other philosophers instead. But the subsequent class discussions would most likely be riveting.

MUSIC

The energies that become manifested as sound are often integral to alternative states of consciousness. In Hinduism one name of the Creator is Nada Brahma, the Sound-God. In ancient Greece, the Pythagoreans, who excelled in their comprehension of mathematics, also wrote about "the music of the spheres." Whether Pythagoras of Samos personally ingested entheogenic substances somewhere around 500 BCE or whether he was a natural mystic who encountered mystical realms in other ways, we have no way of knowing. Even in relative silence, people often report hearing music in other states of awareness. The Sufi mystic Hazrat Inayat Khan taught that ultimately the universe is made up of vibrations that he called music. In his devotion, he believed he actually became music: "I played the vina until my heart turned into the same instrument. Then I offered this instrument to the divine Musician, the only musician existing. Since then I have become His flute, and when He chooses He plays His music. The people give me credit for this music which, in reality, is not due to me, but to the Musician who plays on His own instrument."

When listening to music during the action of entheogens, it is common to hear claims of "having become the music," of "entering into the mind of the composer," or of beholding the eternal truth that the composer was attempting to depict or express in his or her composition. Music is thus often understood to be a nonverbal language that seeks to express, and is indeed capable of expressing, the deepest processes and ultimate truths within human consciousness. As illustrated by a Brahms symphony, for example, this includes not only the richly expressive harmonies, but also the often-dissonant diminished and augmented chord progressions that rise and fall before eventually reaching a climax. As lovers of classical music know well, this is often felt to parallel the struggles and joys of human existence, musical forms that tap into our deepest yearnings and most sacred intuitions.

Thus, it is reasonable to conclude that "getting inside the music" as opposed to objectively listening to music from a critical distance with the categories of the rational mind and language in full swing is almost guaranteed to be of significant value for many scholars of music, performers, and composers. It might well enhance the ability to grasp "what the composer was trying to say" and it also might catalyze one's own ability to translate the depths of one's own being into new compositions. Hearing a recording such as Leopold Stokowski's arrangement of J. S. Bach's "Come Sweet Death" with the expanded awareness provided by the use of an entheogen, for example, may trigger profound appreciation for the art of Stokowski in interpreting the music and evoking the expressive potentials within each of the members of his orchestra and for the genius of Bach himself, as well as awe at what some would consider the transcendental beauty tenderly emanating from eternal realms of consciousness to those of us who are listening in the world of time. Music we call "great," often classical, choral, or symphonic, is also repeatedly claimed by some to be "the language of the gods." There are alternative states of consciousness in which music is intuitively known to reflect and express spiritual truth far above and beyond the threshold where words falter and cease.

We often marvel at genius in music–how Beethoven composed and directed his triumphant Ninth Symphony when he was deaf, or how Handel penned his oratorio, *Messiah*, in only about twenty-four days. The exquisite pathos and exultant glory of Brahms's German Requiem, the magnificence of J. S. Bach's Mass in B Minor, or the transcendental yearnings and ethereal climax of Samuel Barber's Adagio for Strings (also popularly known as the "Theme Song from *Platoon*") are intuitively recognized as profoundly spiritual by many listeners. More recently, we have marvelous compositions, often considered mystical, by such composers as Olivier Messiaen, Henryk Górecki, and Arvo Pärt. Messiaen, for example, credited Hindu chant and birdsongs among the sources of works with titles like *Quartet for the End of Time* and *Illuminations on the Beyond*. It is reasonable to hypothesize that music that reaches so deeply into the human soul arose in profoundly sacred alternative states of consciousness, regardless of how they may have been engendered.

The use of entheogens by musicians has also produced a variety of experimental compositions, often catalogued under categories like psychedelic rock, soul, folk, and pop, as well as electronic music called trance or rave. Some may seem to reflect more superficial changes in consciousness, perhaps a manifestation of alternative states of sensory change and delightful displays of color and geometric forms; others appear to probe more deeply into the mind where experiences commonly considered sacred are to be encountered. Some intricate percussive music, such as the trance music of Abdelmadjid Guemguem, known as Guem, has been reported to catalyze profoundly spiritual states of awareness for some listeners. Also, the use of psychedelic substances for many has triggered a newfound appreciation for classical Indian ragas, such as the Carnatic compositions of Tyagaraja (1767–1847), with their repetitive rhythms and quarter-tone pitches. Even solemn Gregorian chants, mantras that often catalyze the progressive deepening of meditative forms of awareness, have been found uniquely effective by some people. After several decades of experimenting with the choice of many different styles of music to provide nonverbal support during the action of psychedelic substances, trying to differentiate between the "very good" and the "excellent," I have personally concluded that there are works by Bach, Brahms, Mozart, and other composers usually considered "Western classical" that definitely qualify as "supremely psychedelic."

I vividly recall an evening in the mountainous terrain of Northern India, when I had been graciously invited to dinner in the home of Tendzin Choegyal and his wife, Rinchen Khandro. Tendzin was born a Tulku, but had chosen to disengage from his monastic lineage, marry, and have children. He is also the youngest brother of Tenzin Gyatso, His Holiness, the 14th Dalai Lama. Rinchen, a most remarkable woman, is the founder and director of the Tibetan Nuns Project, a compassionate, nonprofit, educational endeavor that, on several small, beautifully designed campuses, houses and supports some seven hundred women refugees who are adjusting to life in India. Their home, just below the Dalai Lama's compound, is located on a steep hillside, high above the valley below and the town of Dharamsala. Adding to the exotic magic of the scene that evening were several magnificent eagles, gracefully soaring and swooping through the sky.

Feeling honored to be in the presence of these auspicious Tibetan leaders for a few precious hours, I asked myself what I most wanted to discuss with them. One topic my mind seized upon was Tibetan music with its orchestration of unique horns, drums, cymbals, and gongs. I had heard of theories that different piercing or reverberating frequencies of sound might evoke various discrete phenomena within human consciousness and had listened to monks gutturally chanting "om mani padme hum" (roughly, "homage to the jewel in the center of the lotus") in the temple of the Dalai Lama with occasional bursts of instrumental accompaniment. "Tendzin," I said, "I'd be interested to learn something from you about Tibetan music and its relationship to consciousness." After a calming pause, he smiled and answered, "Bill, if you want to know the music that moves me most deeply spiritually, it is Beethoven's Pastoral Symphony."

Hanscarl Leuner, who developed a psychotherapeutic technique known as Guided Affective Imagery, or GAI (Experimentelles katatymes Bilderleben, or EkB), may be credited as being the first to combine imagery with music and then to combine both with the use of entheogens. His techniques, combined with the experiences of others who employed music in the early days of psychedelic research in Canada, the United States, and Europe, were further refined and systematized by Helen Lindquist Bonny, a music therapist at the Maryland Psychiatric Research Center. Her seminal work has become known as the Bonny Method of Guided Imagery and Music (GIM) and continues to be applied, usually without entheogens, in many countries associated with the Association for Music and Imagery (www.ami-bonnymethod.org).

Similarly, Stanislav Grof has combined these techniques with an emphasis on focused, rapid breathing that he named "Holotropic Breathwork," now widely disseminated and centrally organized through the Association for Holotropic Breathwork International (www.grof-holotropic-breathwork.net). Both Helen Bonny and Stan Grof have also utilized an art therapy technique of drawing mandalas, developed by Joan Kellogg, that was employed in psychedelic research at the Maryland Psychiatric Research Center to facilitate the initial expression and integration of psychedelic experiences. For musicians interested in joining this creative ferment of facilitating psychotherapeutic processes with the adjunctive use of mental imagery procedures, breathing techniques, and artistic expression, with or without the use of entheogens, the research opportunities are extensive. In future psychotherapy research with various entheogens, a comparison or control group could be offered treatment with Guided Affective Imagery, Guided Imagery with Music, or Holotropic Breathwork.

There are musicians who, in search of unique perspectives and inspiration, choose to take the risks of unauthorized psychedelic use, coping with the uncertainties of purity and dosage of whatever natural or synthetic substances may be available through illicit channels of distribution while taking responsibility for their decision to violate the current drug laws. Impatient to live their lives and compose while they can, they may have concluded that it is highly improbable that college seminars or professional workshops that include legal entheogenic exploration will become available during their productive years. I would encourage such musicians to collaborate with social scientists and medical professionals in the design and implementation of culturally sanctioned research projects with psychedelic substances, now in the present time, in hopes of paving the way for legal access to entheogens in well-structured settings, perhaps for themselves, but certainly for composers and performers in the future.

LITERATURE

The unfolding story lines of many novels that we view as reflecting greatness appear to arise deep within the minds of their authors. The dreamlike sequences that an author may imagine in his or her own inner field of consciousness and subsequently express in writing are very similar, if not identical, with the flow of content that occurs in some psychedelic sessions. Intricate dramas are often woven or choreographed by some ingenious part of our minds that skillfully dramatizes the unfolding of our personal psychological and spiritual lives, often including themes that are relevant to others who are living through the same emotional tensions or period of history. Many of these dramas, sometimes called myths in the making, include a rich variety of human emotions, moments sometimes profoundly serious, even earth-shaking, and also sometimes playful and humorous.

When one reads classics such as Dante's *Divine Comedy*, Milton's *Paradise Lost*, Bunyan's *Pilgrim's Progress*, or even Hesse's *Siddhartha* with memories of one's own visionary or mystical experiences in the background, it is easy to appreciate "where the author is coming from." The crafting of such stories with words may be recognized as the art of communicating insights about ultimate meanings in life and as attempts to guide readers to similar discoveries as their own conflicts, emotions, and yearnings resonate with the characters in the novels. Some of these works come to be considered classics and endure from one generation to the next precisely because they tap into universal, perhaps mystical principles in the human mind.

Poems, especially, sometimes appear to arise out of the struggle to give expression with carefully selected words and their associations to experiences that are often felt to elude precise linguistic formulation. The element of surprise during the sequences of imagery in many psychedelic sessions parallels the unanticipated twists and turns in the plots of many fine novels. Someday, perhaps there will be optional weekend retreats associated with courses in creative writing where some motivated students, safely and legally, deeply can explore their imaginal processes with the facilitation of entheogens.

NEUROSCIENCE

What experiential knowledge, or at least clues by which to formulate fresh hypotheses, might await people skilled in such disciplines as biochemistry, neuroanatomy, cellular biology, or quantum physics? Claims have long been made of the value of psychedelic substances in facilitating creativity. To formulate and test new hypotheses, one, of course, must have done his or her homework and mastered the language and current conceptual frameworks of a particular academic discipline. This is one reason that the prospect of psychedelic substances being made legally available to mature scholars tends to evoke excitement and hope.

A beginning in the exploration of this use of psychedelics occurred in Menlo Park, California, in the late 1960s in a study of creativity, as reported in the book by James Fadiman *The Psychedelic Explorer's Guide.* Participants were respected and well established in their disciplines, could articulate an unsolved problem or issue on the growing edge of their fields, and then were presented with their chosen topic during the latter hours of a psychedelic session, usually with LSD. Many claimed to be able to view their impasses or frontiers from new perspectives, to explore the interrelationships between ideas, to uniquely visualize and obtain insights, some of which became manifested in practical, completed projects afterward.

If, from at least one perspective, we not only have nerves but indeed *are* nerves, one cannot help but wonder what experiential knowledge might await well-trained neuroscientists who are given the opportunity to explore their own nervous systems with the assistance of entheogens. As noted earlier, Jeremy Narby, though an anthropologist, in his book *The Cosmic Serpent: DNA and the Origins of Knowledge*, has offered a fascinating suggestion. He posits that, just as we have externally oriented senses that provide us with visual, auditory, olfactory, cutaneous, and kinesthetic reception, we may also have an internally oriented ability to perceive neuronal, cellular, and perhaps genetic structures and processes. He calls attention to the colorful, abstract patterns and geometrical designs often reported during the action of entheogens and boldly suggests that in these visions we may actually be perceiving atomic and subatomic substrates of our own nervous systems. He notes that DNA purportedly emits light in the form of photons and posits that at times during psychedelic sessions people may actually be seeing DNA spirals and similar phenomena. Of course, it is easy to dismiss Narby's speculation and label it as schizoid. But can any of us posit an alternative explanation for these inner experiences that are encountered so reliably and that we tend to find so impressive and convincing?

Similarly, the psychiatrist Rick Strassman in his book *DMT: The Spirit Molecule* invites researchers to take a fresh look at the pineal gland, which the philosopher René Descartes, way back in the late sixteenth century and early seventeenth, believed to be the "seat of the soul." Dr. Strassman has posited that DMT may indeed be produced by the pineal gland near the center of each of our brains, just below the back of our corpora callosa, and could conceivably secrete larger-than-usual dosage when near-death, psychotic, or spontane-ous mystical experiences are reported. In 2013 a research study by Steven Barker and colleagues provided initial confirmation of DMT in the microdialysis of rat pineal tissue, marking the beginning of a trail that awaits biochemists interested in further explorations. Whether or not future research will support the hypothesis that our brains indeed produce endogenous DMT, there are reports that it is naturally gener-ated somewhere in our bodies, perhaps in lung tissue, and that trace amounts have been found in human blood and urine. This invites spec-ulation about the role of DMT in life and evolution in general, as it is reportedly found throughout the animal and plant kingdoms. It also invites the rather amusing thought that, with possession of DMT for-bidden by many governments at this point in history, most of us by vir-tue of being human may unwittingly be in violation of federal law even if the quantity of the entheogen in our bodies is usually miniscule. This suggestion is easily discounted since the amount of DMT measured is often barely detectable; yet we know that LSD can be psychoactive in doses as low as twenty millionths of a gram.

BOTANY

A frequently reported change in the way life is viewed after profound psychedelic experiences is enhanced appreciation for intelligence in nature. Plants, trees, animals, birds, and even mushroom mycelia and bacteria begin to be viewed and respected as autonomous living beings, rather than simply as mindless or mechanical objects in our environment awaiting exploitation or control for the convenience of the human species. Darwin's interpretation of evolution as "survival of the fittest," as discussed in books by Jeremy Narby, Michael Pollan, and Simon Powell, is becoming tempered by a recognition of and apprecia-tion for ingeniously clever forms of behavior that appear to reflect not only adaptation but learning.

Increasingly researchers are discovering the presence of DMT in significant concentrations in various plant species, some that have long been valued as medicines and that have been ritually employed by indigenous shamans or healers. In the sacred brew called ayahuasca, it is usually the leaves of the plant *Psychotria veridis*, also called Chacruna, that contain DMT. Ingested alone, the leaves are orally inactive due to the inhibiting action of monoamine oxidase enzymes in the human stomach. However, when combined with the MAO-inhibitors harmine, harmaline, and tetrahydroharmine obtained from crushing the vine *Bannesteriopsis caapi*, a liana that rapidly climbs and produces pink blossoms in the crowns of trees, the DMT-containing brew is able to retain its potency and become absorbed in the human body. This facilitates the occurrence of the alternative states of consciousness valued in South American religions, such as the Santo Daime, the União do Vegetal, and the Barquina. In a very similar brew, usually called yagé, the leaves of another DMT-containing plant, *Diplopterys cabrerana*, are combined with the same vine. When asked how the native shamans ever discovered this combination, the answer usually offered is that the plants themselves or the plant spirits taught them the secret.

Belief in "plant teachers" is a troubling and confusing concept—if not pure nonsense—for most of us who have grown up in societies unaccustomed to being receptive to intuitive insights in alternative states of awareness. We may have heard of lonely little old ladies who talk to their plants and perhaps some of us have managed to respond with bemused condescending kindness, but it wouldn't occur to most of us to take their claims seriously, no matter how healthy and robust their plants may appear to be. Even more extreme, there are those who genuinely believe that plants and fungi not only may in some sense be conscious, but also may be capable of intention. Some would see them as reaching out to humanity, perhaps in an effort to sufficiently awaken us to the spiritual dimension of life so that we may not destroy ourselves and our planet by our ecological blindness and unfettered exploitation of natural resources.

We have been taught that problem solving requires brains, preferably human ones. Research reports indicating that unicellular slime molds that don't even have nervous systems can navigate mazes, as discussed by Jeremy Narby in *Intelligence in Nature*, are simply hard to believe no matter how often the experiment is replicated.

One of the ways Edmund Ware Sinnott, for many years chairman of the biology department at Yale University, referred to God was as "the purposive properties of protoplasm." In his books, such as *The Biology of the Spirit* and *Matter, Mind and Man*, he wrote not only about photosynthesis and cellular structures, but also about Beauty and The Divine Spirit. A beginning in bridging this conceptual gap may be found in reverence and purely aesthetic appreciation of beauty and purposive activity in nature, such as has been captured in the incredible time-lapse and time-accelerating photography of Louis Schwartzberg (Movingart.com).

In his book *Mycelium Running*, Paul Stamets, a well-respected mycologist, describes *Psilocybe cubensis*, one of the approximately 180 different species of psilocybin-containing mushrooms, and then comments as follows:

> Currently the cultivation of this mushroom is illegal in the United States, but it is legal in many other countries. . . . However, the legal status of this mushroom and other psychoactive *Psilocybe* species is often in a state of flux as governments struggle with legal definitions. Consult the appropriate legal statutes before pursuing cultivation.
>
> I do not recommend this mushroom for use by the general public. However, in my opinion, this species and its relatives can be helpful for sparking creativity in artists, philosophers, theologians, mathematicians, physicists, astronomers, computer programmers, psychologists, and other intellectual leaders.
>
> I personally believe that the computer and internet industries and astrophysics have been inspired through use of this fungus, which has stimulated the imagination and fields of vision of scientists and shamans with complex fractals, hyperlinking of thoughts and mental tools for complex systems analysis. Many users over thousands of years have elevated this and other *Psilocybe* mushrooms to the level of a religious sacrament.

Perhaps botanists, if not biologists in general, should be added to Stamet's list of those for whom an entheogenic experience may spark creativity. It appears that there may indeed be ways of meaningfully interacting with and learning from certain species of plants and fungi that may facilitate knowledge and appreciation not currently available in most textbooks. Simon G. Powell artfully expressed some of these insights in his film *Manna–Psilocybin Mushroom Inspired Documentary*, released in 2003. Yet it should be noted that, while the first edition of Stamet's book was being printed, the possession of fresh mushrooms containing psilocybin was declared illegal in the United Kingdom in the Drug Act of 2005. The legality of possession, sale, transport, and cultivation of both fresh and dried species of mushrooms containing psilocybin in many countries remains in flux.

CONCLUDING COMMENTS

These psychedelic frontiers in education, notably in philosophy, music, literature, neuroscience, and botany, have been selected more or less at random. It is probable that there is knowledge to be found in entheogenic experiences that is relevant to many other disciplines as well. There have been claims of psychedelic experiences catalyzing creativity in Silicon Valley, especially in the field of computer science. Physicists and mathematicians might well discover many new insights. The relevance of entheogens for religious scholarship will be explored in the following chapter.

I reiterate that these sacred substances are incredibly potent and need to be integrated into education with wisdom and skill. As will be discussed in chapter 16, there are some people for whom the ingestion of entheogens may entail significant risks. Yet to attempt to render them inaccessible and to declare their use illegal for all citizens simply doesn't make sense to those who understand their promise and have learned how to use them responsibly.

15

Psychedelic Frontiers
in Religion

EMPIRICAL EXPERIENCE IN RELIGIOUS SCHOLARSHIP

The world of religious scholarship often seems quite far removed from the world of private devotion and faith, sometimes with heavy reliance on intellectual processes and minimal regard for the intuitive matters of the heart and the experiential domains of the religious life. This scholarly disconnection struck me most poignantly during the final year of my theological studies at the Yale Divinity School, the year after I returned from the University of Göttingen. In Germany, I had attended lectures offered by seminal biblical scholars, including such luminaries as Joachim Jeremias, Hans Conzelmann, and Walther Zimmerli, to the envy of some of my fellow classmates at Yale. Yet strangely enough, I found my primary intellectual yearnings and spiritual inspiration nourished in lectures not in the theological division of the university, but by members of the psychiatric faculty in the School of Medicine. There I found courses such as *Religionspsychopathologie* (the psychopathology of religion) and a seminar on the religious delusions of schizophrenic patients that explored whether or not there were religious revelations that should not be considered evidence of mental illness. The conclusion was that there indeed were such experiences. There was also a course in self-hypnosis and meditative procedures (Schultz's "Autogenic Training") taught in a large auditorium filled primarily with medical students. Coupled with my personal experiences and internship opportunities with psychedelic substances in the psychiatric clinic with Hanscarl Leuner, it was clear to me that I had discovered the experiential dimension of religion being most intensely manifested in the medical division of the university. So it was that, when I returned to New Haven to complete the third and final year of the master of divinity degree, the area of specialization in which I felt most at home had changed from preparation for the pastoral ministry to what then was called "Teaching and Research in Religion."

Back at Yale, one of the first seminars in which I enrolled was titled "The Theology of German Idealism." It focused on writings of the philosophers Kant, Hegel, and Schelling and met around a heavy oak table in the Gothic Sterling Library with windows of tinted stained glass and oil paintings in elaborate gold frames of somber professors wearing academic robes who seemed to be looking down on us. As was the tradition then among graduate students of philosophy, who liked to think of themselves as quite independent, most all students wore tweed sport coats with leather patches on the elbows, rather wrinkled dress shirts with long ties, and denim blue jeans. This was in 1964, and serious philosophers also smoked pipes then, usually curved ones. Further, it was basically a men's club and most everyone was bearded.

I vividly recall the day when, after reading that best seller by Immanuel Kant, titled *The Critique of Pure Reason*, we were seriously pondering a concept of Kant's that he called "intellectual intuition," debating whether or not it was possible directly to know spiritual truth. Kant himself tended to think it was not possible. Fresh from a visit to Baltimore's Spring Grove Hospital, where alcoholics were receiving psychotherapy assisted by LSD under a grant from the National Institute of Mental Health, I found myself remembering a conversation with a man who had suffered from alcoholism, had been hospitalized, and had experienced a mystical form of consciousness during the action of LSD.

I was wearing a traditional tweed sport coat, dress shirt, and tie but, alas, had no leather patches on my elbows. Worse than that, I neither smoked a pipe nor had grown a beard. Nonetheless, I summoned the courage to raise my hand and say something like, "Well, I just visited a research center in Baltimore and spoke with an alcoholic who reported a mystical experience with LSD, and he said, 'Yes, it is possible directly to know spiritual truth.'" A stunned, very awkward silence followed, as if I had violated a sacred academic taboo by introducing empirical information into a philosophical discussion. Time momentarily seemed to have stopped. Then, without anyone responding to my words, the drone resumed and debate continued with selected references to the writings of philosophers long dead whether such knowledge could be possible. It seemed incomprehensible that sophisticated Yale graduate students could learn anything from some alcoholic who had taken a drug.

Psychedelic substances are powerfully effective tools in the study of consciousness, and especially in the study of religious and mystical experiences. If understanding topics like conversion and revelation, and perhaps even the primal origin of religious ideas and sacred symbols, is relevant to religious scholars, why are university departments of religion not collaborating with colleagues who possess research skills in psychopharmacology and seeking the governmental and institutional authorizations currently required to pursue studies with entheogens? Would astronomers be content to pursue research without telescopes, or biologists without microscopes? Or, as mentioned earlier, would a scholar of life in Paris be content to remain within the confines of his college library, mastering the French language and reading French novels and guidebooks without ever walking the streets of the city, speaking with natives in sidewalk cafes, and experiencing the glories of the cathedrals there? Perhaps it is still too early, and religious scholars are just beginning to awaken from a long sleep to the incredible frontier that awaits them. Sociologists are known to have accused religious scholars as suffering from "cultural lag."

Astronomers must sometimes tremble with awe when they look through their telescopes and behold the unfathomable beauty of distant galaxies, but they still manage to formulate hypotheses and make careful observations and measurements in advancing their field of knowledge. The same could be true of religious scholars who genuinely would like to better understand the "mind of God" and the mysteries of our own being. I do not believe that anything sacred would be profaned in such study; if anything, we might discover that areas of life and thought we may have considered profane are indeed being made sacred.

UNDERDEVELOPED AREAS OF RELIGIOUS THOUGHT

There are many exciting frontiers of thought awaiting further exploration by religious scholars. Wayne Teasdale, author of *The Mystic Heart*, one of the finest introductions to mysticism and the meditative life, was a pioneer in interrelating Christianity and Buddhism. Another visionary pioneer is Diana Eck, professor of comparative religion at Harvard, who has been building bridges of understanding between Christianity and Hinduism—for example, relating the Hindu concept of divine energy called Shakti to the Christian concept of the Holy Spirit. Huston Smith's classic survey of world religions, *The World's Religions* (titled in earlier editions *The Religions of Man*), reflects his profound appreciation of each of the great faiths, and is written from "within looking out" on the bases of his open-minded immersion in different realms of religious thought and practice as well as his warm personal relationships with leaders from varied religious heritages. Alan Watts, Jack Kornfield, Joseph Goldstein, and others have helped to make Buddhism accessible to Western minds. There is much to be learned from the study of each of the great world religions, and now study need not be limited to the scrutiny of ancient texts but also, with the wise use of psychedelic substances, could be approached within conscious experiencing. As one of many examples, I often think how those Jews, Christians, and Muslims who tend to be excessively serious and somber, if not dour, could benefit from the Hindu appreciation for *lila*, known as "divine playfulness."

There was a time, not long ago, when many scholars of mysticism differentiated between "Eastern Mysticism" with its emphasis on unitive consciousness and "Western Mysticism" with its focus on the personal relationship with the Divine. Now, as discussed earlier, we know that many, if not most, people, Eastern or Western, can experience both of these forms of consciousness. Similarly, as discussed in the chapter on "Approaches to Unitive Consciousness," it now appears that both "Internal Unity" and "External Unity," far from representing two different cultures or ways in which nervous systems may function, appear to be potential experiences within the repertoire of many human beings.

Actually, the breadth of theological scholarship and personal experience within individual religious traditions can often be found to include both unitive consciousness and devotion to the divine in personal manifestations. Hinduism includes not only acknowledgment of the Atman/Brahman unity, but also worship of the Ishwara in forms such as Lord Shiva or Lord Krishna. Christianity spans both the abstract ground of being as described by Paul Tillich and devotion to the personal Jesus. I remember entering a Hindu temple on Krishna's birthday, seeing smiling little children gathered around a crib in which rested a baby Krishna doll, and being struck with how similar it was to the typical manger scenes on Christmas Eve in the Christian tradition. The behavior of altar guild members is delightfully similar, whether polishing brass crosses, candlesticks, water bowls, or statues of different deities. While theological distinctions can always be made and valued, there is ample room to find meaningful similarities and connections within the faiths of the world, and perhaps to unite in projects of social service.

There are many theological phrases and concepts that can become illumined with new understandings. For example, consider the oft-quoted scripture from Exodus (33:20), "You cannot see God and live." It would be easy to dismiss such an idea as simply wrong on the basis of the many people who indeed feel they have "seen God" and obviously are still alive. Yet many of them have experienced a death of the ego, or everyday self, in conjunction with the revelation of the eternal world, and in that sense were indeed "dead" when the visionary world manifested itself. Similarly, St. Paul wrote of "dying to self" in the process of becoming a "new being in Christ." This invites clarification of language and provides opportunities for fresh theological reflections.

Thomas Roberts has written about the "five hundred year old blizzard of words," triggered by the invention of the printing press and the access of the common man to sacred scriptures and theological commentaries. He now foresees a new religious era with less reliance on words and greater emphasis on direct primary religious experiences, and has written, "To most people who are even moderately experienced with entheogens, concepts such as awe, sacredness, eternity, grace, agape, transcendence, transfiguration, dark night of the soul, born- again, heaven and hell are more than theological ideas; they are experiences." Such experiential understanding of religious concepts need not devalue traditional creeds and dogma, but can infuse symbolic language with new meaning, rendering it more accessible and comprehensible to those of us who now worship in the twenty-first century.

In regard to the theological concept of "sin," entheogenic experiences tend to support movement away from a legalistic list of specific prohibited attitudes or acts toward an understanding of sin as estrangement or separation from the Divine. Entering into the world of time thus entails "original sin" as separation, though not necessarily as "fallen" or guilt-ridden. Matthew Fox is one theologian who has written about this new perspective, calling attention to what he called "Original Blessing." Paul Tillich has similarly invited us to consider sin as estrangement from ourselves, one another, and the Ground of Being. Redemption or salvation, in contrast, may be seen as reestablishing a conscious connection with the sacred dimensions of consciousness.

Religious symbols can undergo a metamorphosis from intellectual concepts to spiritual realities bursting with significance. This is perhaps supremely manifested in the Roman Catholic doctrine of transubstantiation, in which the wine and bread of the communion elements may be spiritually experienced as the blood and body of the Christ and all the profound meanings that the symbols of "blood" and "body" can portray. Without deciphering the symbols, especially for those who have not grown up within a Christian tradition, the ritual of the mass may simply appear strange and bizarre, as if drinking blood and eating flesh were some primitive cannibalistic practice that unthinking modern men and women continue to reenact for unknown reasons. With more attunement to the spiritual dimension of life, there can be enhanced appreciation of the mysteries within the Eucharistic symbols, of the altar as a focal location in time and space where eternal verities and temporal existence may meet and where genuine spiritual nourishment may be obtained. Blood in particular appears to be a symbol often encountered in psychedelic experiences, not as something gory, but as a cleansing, vibrantly red, life-giving energy in the visionary world; this makes sense of the common religious phrase in the Judeo-Christian tradition "washed in the blood of the lamb."

UNDERSTANDING PROPHETS AND PROPHECY

Religious scholars tend to view prophets not primarily as "fore-tellers" but as "forth-tellers." In the sacred scriptures of Judaism, Christianity, and Islam, there are many descriptions of visionary or archetypal experiences. In the wake of such revelations, prophets inspired by the alternative states of consciousness they experienced, such as Amos, Hosea, Isaiah, Ezekiel, Jeremiah, Zechariah, Zephaniah, and Muhammad, typically preached about the need for spiritual awakening, renewed ethical standards, and the importance of social justice. From an Islamic perspective, Isa, or Jesus of Nazareth, would be included in the list. Many of the descriptions of visionary experiences, expressed by these men or attributed to them, also stress the exalted, primary reality of God, utter humility in the divine presence, the potency of love and wrath, the reality of death, and the brevity of human life.

Would it be too radical to suggest that a similar visionary experience might prove instructive to a scholar of sacred scriptures? Rick Strassman in his book *DMT and the Soul of Prophecy* has provided an initial impetus in this direction with his comparison of some of the DMT experiences reported by his subjects and writings by, or carrying the name of, the Hebrew prophets. Scholars have often focused on the meanings of the scriptural words in their original languages and have sought to reconstruct the historical, social, and political periods in which the prophets lived. In addition, experiential appreciation for the visionary realms that the prophets encountered could provide new vitality in religious studies.

Various religions in the world have focused on a single prophetic voice, a written document, or a collection of manuscripts and claimed it to be the final revelation of God to man. With due respect for individual systems of belief, it is clear that, though one may choose a definitive focus that one personally considers sufficient, in actuality revelation continues to occur, not only within particular religions but within human psyches with diverse languages, traditions, and orientations in different cultures of the world. It has been suggested by some who have experienced revelatory states of consciousness that, even if all the scriptures of the world were somehow lost, tragic as that event would be for history and literature as well as religions, in time similar scriptures with similarly profound spiritual insights would come to be written.

Scriptures, no matter how deeply revered, have never fallen out of the skies and hit prophets on their heads; they have always been written by inspired human beings who personally experienced alternate states of awareness in various sociopolitical settings and expressed the revelations they encountered as best they could in speech or writing. Often their followers, sometimes decades later, wrote down stories or poems that had been orally transmitted and edited the manuscripts as best they could. As the histories of organized religions have progressed, committees of scholars have prayerfully assembled to vote on which allegedly inspired manuscripts to include in their official scriptures and which to exclude. As encapsulated in the quotation by Paul Tillich in the frontispiece of this book, "God has not left himself unwitnessed."

THE POWER OF DECISIONS

Among the experiential learnings for religious scholars who could pursue research with psychedelic substances would be a clearer understanding of the role of choice or decision in religious lives. Evangelical Protestantism has especially emphasized the "decision for Christ," an active act of choosing to be receptive, to entrust one's self to something greater than one's everyday personality, and to allow a sacred dimension of life, however conceptualized, to enter, change, and transform one's being. This moment or process of awakening usually requires more than the passivity symbolized by listlessly lying on pavement while a steamroller approaches. Viewed from a psychological perspective, this also acknowledges the importance of ego-strength, how when one "has an ego" or some sense of a developed personal identity, it becomes easier under the right conditions to choose to relinquish ego controls. Perhaps this is why people in their mid-twenties and beyond may be more likely to experience transcendental states of consciousness during the action of entheogens than younger people amid the

turmoil of adolescence. Yet, in view of the frequency with which conversion experiences spontaneously occur in many young adolescents
in the contexts of evangelical religious groups, it would appear that
some teenagers already possess an adequately strong sense of identity
or selfhood.

IN AND OUT OF THEOLOGICAL CIRCLES

In the process of interrelating my own Christian theological education and studies of world religions with the experiential knowledge
derived from mystical and archetypal experiences, a conceptual tool I
have found of significant value is Paul Tillich's idea of the "theological
circle." Within the confines of a circle, one is immersed in the symbol-
ism, language, and historical traditions of one's religious faith, be it
Christian, Hindu, or any of the other world religions. One feels the
meanings and senses the dramas portrayed within the particular faith
tradition and can thus enter into worship or meditative experiences as
a full participant.

However, one can also at times step outside the circle, empowering
the rational minds of the philosopher and scientist within us all. From
this perspective, one can critically examine the contents within a particular circle and also relate and compare one circle with another. With
sufficient training, one can even enter fully into a circle different from
one's childhood religion or culture. Here is a very practical application
of the "Both/And" orientation that honors both the cognitive and the
intuitive capacities with which we have been endowed. Scholars of
religion need not be skeptical agnostics who always maintain a critical
distance from their subject matter. Nor need they be so myopically
focused on one particular religion that they ignore or devalue others.
In this particular discipline, perhaps more than many others, the very
essence of one's being is involved in one's area of study and one can
both worship and think.

As one who values being a participant observer in religious traditions different from my own heritage, I recall praying at the Wailing
Wall in the Old City of Jerusalem. Once my prayers were completed,
as I walked the ascending pathway that led away from the wall, I saw
an orthodox rabbi approaching me in a black robe with a very long

white beard, sparkling eyes, and a warm smile. I looked forward to interacting with him and perhaps, however briefly, sharing something of our lives and mutual perspectives. He grasped my hands and looked me straight in the eye as we greeted each other. Then, he paused and slowly inquired, "Was your mother Jewish?" When I indicated a negative answer, his response was a very curt "have a good day" while he briskly walked away. Perhaps he was only in search of a tenth member for a minyan for public prayers, but he and I both missed an opportunity to really meet and to perhaps learn from each other.

In another attempt to enter deeply into a somewhat different religious tradition, I confess to having respectfully communed at the high altar of St. Peter's Basilica in Rome even though I am officially a Protestant and had not gone to formal confession before communing as is usually expected in Catholicism. I am happy to report that I was not struck dead. My experiences of meditating in Buddhist, Hindu, and Sikh temples and in Islamic mosques have also been without incident and, frankly, I have often found them to be meaningful worship experiences. In the Episcopal parish where I find myself contributing as a musician on most Sunday mornings, I'm aware of sometimes entering into the circle of Christian dogmatics sufficiently to meaningfully recite and mentally decipher the historic Nicene Creed, even including the symbolic language "He ascended into heaven and is seated at the right hand of the Father." At other times I discover that I have stepped outside the circle and, though still genuinely worshiping, am meditatively immersed privately in a Hindu or Buddhist chant.

THE JESUS OF HISTORY AND THE ETERNAL CHRIST

It was Carl Jung who posited that the archetype of the Christ is to be found within us all, irrespective of whether we grew up as Christians or whether we consider ourselves "believers." The German theologian Martin Kähler is noted for making a distinction between the Jesus of history and the Christ of faith—the latter being the eternal archetype who always has been and who was before the birth of the historical man called Jesus of Nazareth and of course continued to be after his crucifixion. Within this framework of understanding, the eternal Christ dwells within each human being, regardless of religious or nonreligious systems of personal belief, and, as with Saul of Tarsus, who became St. Paul, may reveal himself in visionary experiences. This may also prove to be true of other major archetypes, including the Buddha and bodhisattvas, Hindu deities, Greek gods, and what Jung called "The Wise Old Man," The Child," and "The Great Mother." If this proves to be validated by empirical research studies in the future, it may not be considered unusual for a Hindu to encounter the Christ or for a Christian to encounter Shiva or Vishnu.

INQUIRY INTO THE ORIGINS OF RELIGIONS

For scholars interested in pursuing the possible role of entheogens in the origin of religions, there are intriguing frontiers to explore. Carefully researched books have been published by authors such as Robert Gordon Wasson, Huston Smith, Carl Ruck, Albert Hofmann, and Dan Merkur, suggesting that the *soma* described in the ancient Rig Veda, the *kykeon* drunk in the Eleusinian Mystery religions, and even the *manna* that the Israelites harvested in the early morning en route to Canaan may well have been species of psychoactive mushrooms. The archeologist and scholar of the Dead Sea Scrolls John Marco Allegro, in his book *The Sacred Mushroom and the Cross*, generated intense controversy by suggesting that references to Jesus in the Gospels may have been a code for the potentially sacred effects of a mushroom, *Amanita muscaria*, and the realms of spiritual knowledge thereby accessed. It is reported that, sensing the difficulties that many theologians would encounter in trying to understand his finding, he resigned from his position on the theological faculty of the University of Manchester when his book was published. Though he died in 1988, some of his insights, as well as those of other scholars, may well merit the careful continuing attention of those who possess the necessary knowledge to decipher ancient documents along with the courageous openness to seriously explore new perspectives.

ENTHEOGENS IN PERSONAL RELIGIOUS PRACTICE

If we turn from the world of scholarship to the personal practice of religion, the emerging cache of knowledge regarding the potential of entheogens, when wisely ingested, to nurture the spiritual awareness of those of us who desire experiential knowledge in our religious lives raises very practical questions. Clearly there are important issues that require discussion and resolution in medical, legal, and religious communities in the near future.

Many would assert that the freedom of religion enshrined by the Constitution of the United States and similar guarantees in other countries must eventually prevail over the cultural fears, fueled by governments who have attempted to suppress and control access to psychedelic substances in either their pharmacologically pure or their plant-based forms. When future historians look back on our era, I suspect they will find it hard to believe, if not totally ludicrous, that fears of consciousness exploration and religious experiences could ever have been so extremely out of control that a person could be subject to arrest if the wrong species of mushroom happened to sprout in his or her yard and especially if one should personally decide to consume it as a sacrament.

At the time of writing, it can be stated that the religious use of mescaline in the form of the Peyote cactus was declared legal in the United States in 1971 for members of the Native American Church. In addition, the US Supreme Court in 2006 recognized DMT in the brew called ayahuasca as a legitimate and legal sacrament of the União do Vegetal (UDV) religion. Use is currently legal for members of these specific religious organizations according to US federal law, though laws in the individual states may differ. Not surprisingly, the importation of the sacramental substances in the states that allow its presence allegedly remains closely monitored by the Drug Enforcement Administration to ensure that there is no diversion to so-called recreational users.

One may hope that continuing respectful and responsible attitudes toward these sacramental substances will gradually lead to them becoming legally accessible in the United States and elsewhere in other contexts where serious religious intent prevails. Perhaps the next step would be to extend legal authorization to retreat and research centers, staffed by professionals with both medical and religious training, who understand the art of wisely administering these substances to those who wish to receive them. Such centers could also provide individual and group support for the initial integration of psychedelic experiences. Although it may be a long time before psychedelic sacraments are incorporated into worship experiences in the churches, synagogues, mosques, and temples of major religious organizations, present religious leaders from diverse faith backgrounds could be supportive of such centers for research and retreat.

16

Maximizing the Probability of Safety and Benefit

PHYSIOLOGICAL SAFETY

On a foundation of many years of experience in indigenous cultures and in modern psychotherapy suites and medical laboratories, the physiological safety of the major entheogens has been quite firmly established. Various studies over several decades have declared them essentially nontoxic as well as physically nonaddictive. They are not considered drugs of dependence since compulsive drug-seeking is not associated with them. Neither reliable self-administration in animal studies nor any detectable withdrawal syndromes have been observed.

The sensationalistic publicity surrounding the death of a seven-thousand-pound elephant called Tusko in the Oklahoma City Zoo, who in 1962 was given an intramuscular injection of 297,000 mcg of LSD, has finally quieted down. Subsequent investigations concluded that in all probability it was not the LSD, but other medications subsequently administered that caused the elephant's death. And though LSD alone has since been administered allegedly to elephants in equally excessive dosage without causing death, the amount administered in this bizarre story was approximately 660 times the typical high dose of LSD (450 mcg) that would be prescribed for a human volunteer. That this event was ever referenced to attempt to document the alleged dangers of LSD is now in retrospect a thought-provoking indicator of the irrational climate present in that period of our history.

Similarly, at that period in time, in the wake of the Thalidomide tragedies that had resulted in birth defects, it was alleged that LSD might cause chromosome damage. Taking this concern seriously, the staff at the Maryland Psychiatric Research Center conducted a carefully designed FDA-approved study, double-blind and controlled, using pure LSD in collaboration with Joe-Hin Tjio, a biochemist at the National Institutes of Health. Blood samples were obtained from thirty-two subjects who participated in our ongoing psychotherapy research studies before and after LSD administration and were transported to a laboratory in Bethesda, Maryland, for microscopic examination. Also, blood samples were obtained from five black-market users who agreed to take pure LSD at the center as well as from eight normal volunteers and staff members who had received pure LSD in the recent past, including myself. The laboratory technicians did not know which samples were drawn before LSD administration and which were obtained afterward. The results of this study, published in 1969 in the prestigious *Journal of the American Medical Association* (JAMA), stated that "there is no definite evidence that pure LSD damages chromosomes of human lymphocytes in vivo as studied from 72-hour cultures." Yet, again as an indicator of the irrational climate at the time, this study and its results received almost no press coverage and well-meaning antidrug warriors persisted in calling attention to the ephemeral specter of chromosome damage.

In 1971, Norman Dishotsky and his colleagues critically surveyed nine "in vitro" (that is, in test tubes) studies that claimed chromosome breakage after LSD and twenty-one "in vivo" (that is, in living human beings) studies that had reported conflicting results. The scientists concluded that "chromosome damage, when found, was related to the effects of drug abuse in general and not, as initially reported, to LSD alone. We believe that pure LSD ingested in moderate dosages does not produce chromosome damage detectable by available methods." They also addressed allegations that LSD might cause cancer or birth defects and found no credible evidence in their review of the literature, but noted that "while there is no evidence that pure LSD is teratogenic in man, the use of any drug during pregnancy requires that its potential benefits significantly outweigh its potential hazards." Ethical guidelines in research projects with most any drug today would disqualify any pregnant woman from participation as a precautionary measure. Our own review at Johns Hopkins of the literature on major entheogens relevant to issues of safety, published in 2008 (by Johnson, Richards, and Griffiths), arrived at similar conclusions.

Clearly the finding of the apparent physiological safety of pure LSD does not automatically generalize to other major entheogens, either in their pharmacologically pure forms or in their manifestations in natural plants or fungi. Many opportunities for carefully implemented research studies await us to supplement and clarify the findings already in the professional literature. It is conceivable, for example, that some of the 180 or more species of mushrooms that contain psilocybin or some of the ingredients occasionally put into ayahuasca preparations could cause some adverse responses in humans.

There are many unknowns to consider when dealing with substances harvested in nature–for example, one never knows for sure if a raccoon urinated on the mushrooms one is harvesting or not or whether such an event would make any difference. However, in light of the long history of the indigenous use of these sacramental substances in religious ceremonies, it is reasonable to consider it improbable that any acutely toxic compounds are to be found. To circumvent the unknowns of the natural growth of psilocybin-containing mushrooms in the open air, often in pastures on cow dung, some people today, with precise instructions easily found via the Internet, order the mushroom spores online. They then inject the spores into vermiculite and brown rice flour with distilled water in sterile wide-mouth mason jars and grow their own supplies. Although growing psilocybin mushrooms, even in the privacy of one's own home for one's own use, is still illegal and, if apprehended, carries harsh penalties in many parts of the world, ordering and possessing the spores, presumably for microscopic examination, remains legal with few exceptions.

Another concern has focused on what has come to be called "hallucinogen persisting perceptual disorder (HPPD)," more commonly characterized by the term "flashbacks." These perceptual changes, sometimes claimed to constitute a recurrence of drug effects in the days or months after the substance is presumably no longer present in the body, appear to be quite rare. They are welcomed by some people and cause distress in others. In almost two decades of research with psychedelic substances at the Spring Grove Hospital and Maryland Psychiatric Research Center, I am aware of no reports of this phenomenon, perhaps because it wasn't expected and volunteers were not questioned about it during follow-up interviews. Researchers at present are inquiring about the phenomenon, so more definitive information should be available in the near future.

It appears that "flashbacks," though rare if existent at all in well-managed research settings, may be more common among people who frequently use a variety of psychoactive drugs and especially among those who do not administer the substances with religious or psychotherapeutic intent. One theory of their origin often suggested proposes that they are more probable when one is seeking a pleasant experience and unresolved conflicts emerge instead, especially if one seeks to avoid the emotional content awaiting confrontation and expression. A significant psychotherapeutic opportunity is presented and, due to lack of motivation or insufficient therapeutic support, the invitation is essentially rejected. The person typically walks around and talks with open eyes, trying to regain control rather than allowing himself or herself to move though the emerging distress toward resolution and healing. Finally, the drug wears off, but the conflict that has been awakened remains just below the threshold of awareness. Then, when the person is under stress or sleep-deprived, so goes the theory, the material that has been triggered and inadequately confronted is understood to reemerge into conscious awareness, essentially offering a second opportunity to deal with the difficult emotional content within.

Another factor to consider in weighing reports of "flashbacks" is that unusual mental states before taking a psychedelic substance tend to simply be viewed as "unusual experiences," but when they occur afterward, their appearance sometimes, rightly or wrongly, may be attributed to a prior psychedelic experience. Alternative states of consciousness have always been known to occur spontaneously, perhaps triggered in part by our own biochemical and psychological processes. In summary, the available information at this point in time supports the fundamental physiological safety of the major entheogens, especially in their pharmacologically pure forms.

It should be noted that, in the medical screening of volunteers for most ongoing research projects with psychedelic substances, there are criteria for excluding people who may be at greater risk than others. For example, as noted earlier, pregnant women, or women intending to become pregnant in the near future, routinely tend to be screened out, a usual and routine precaution in all psychopharmacological research. Similarly, for a person with an acute cardiovascular condition, the risks entailed might well exceed the potential benefits. If one shouldn't ride a rollercoaster or finds it physically dangerous to encounter intense emotions, it well may be unwise to take an entheogen, though I am aware of no well-documented instances of death from intense emotion alone. Nonetheless, both intense psychological pain and intense joy can be downright exhausting. Elderly terminal cancer patients without severe cardiovascular problems have tolerated emotional expression well; even though weary at the end of the day, they have typically expressed gratitude for the experience as a whole.

Most research projects would screen out anyone with a brain tumor, significant neurological metastases from cancer, or a seizure disorder such as epilepsy, both for ethical reasons in wanting to maximize the probability of benefit when there is the presence of unknown factors and for methodological reasons in wanting to standardize the characteristics of the sample of people being studied. In most contemporary studies there are also strict disqualifying standards for people who consistently produce high blood pressure readings. Initial findings at Hopkins indicate a slight rise in blood pressure for most people during the action of psilocybin, and cardiovascular arousal often rises and falls with the emotions being experienced. Further, due to possible unknown factors, people currently taking antidepressant medications such as Prozac, Zoloft, Celexa, or Paxil, which are understood to bind with the same brain receptors as psychedelics, would be well advised to successfully discontinue those medications if possible and appropriate prior to considering participation in psychedelic research.

These, of course, are the guidelines typically followed in controlled medical investigations, usually in university settings. The standards observed in indigenous religious communities may differ, perhaps posing more risks to some participants, but also providing more flexibility for others who may choose to accept those risks. So far as I know, baseline blood pressure readings are not obtained from church members who receive peyote, psilocybin mushrooms, or ayahuasca in their religious services. Whether or not the current screening procedures in research operations represent an overly cautious determination to ensure maximum safety, along with the necessity of reassuring concerned medical colleagues and members of Institutional Review Boards, will become clear in time with increased experience and the accumulation of more substantial caches of data. Most current researchers who are working with psychedelic substances would rather err on the side of being overly cautious, even overprotective, than risk any potentially adverse event that might conceivably necessitate pausing or halting research while investigations are conducted. Although these policies are sometimes very disappointing to highly motivated research volunteers who apply to participate in various studies with entheogens, at this time in history they tend to be considered prudent and necessary.

PSYCHOLOGICAL SAFETY

The psychological safety of entheogen use requires a more complex answer since it depends both upon who the person about to receive the psychedelic substance happens to be and upon the knowledge and skills of the people who may administer the substance and who are present to provide companionship and support as may be needed.

With our present knowledge, anyone with a family or personal history of psychosis would be wise to opt for methods of personal and spiritual growth that do not include entheogens. There appears to be a significant risk for such people that an entheogen may trigger the onset of a prolonged reaction, that is, of unwanted alternative states of consciousness that continue for days or months after the psychedelic substance would normally have been metabolized, thereby returning the person to the baseline awareness of everyday life. For people without genetic tendencies toward psychosis, this risk appears to be minimal and perhaps nonexistent. In a survey of investigations that included a total of twelve hundred research volunteers who had received either LSD or mescaline, none of them classified as "patients," the psychiatrist Sidney Cohen found only one report of alternative states of consciousness lasting more than forty-eight hours. This person turned out to have been the identical twin of a schizophrenic patient who, in most research programs today, would have been excluded during the initial medical evaluation.

Insofar as entheogens may trigger or accelerate the onset of psychosis in people who are already genetically vulnerable, it has been suggested that in time these same people might well manifest psychotic symptoms even if they do not ingest these substances. Thus, it has been reasoned that a psychedelic experience might speed up their entry into treatment or even prevent psychosis by addressing conflicts that have been intensifying over time or by the therapeutic cultivation of increased ego-strength. This raises fundamental questions about timing, motivation, values, and how one conceptualizes the purpose of human life. Is one's goal to "remain normal" or is it to struggle with and through one's conflicts in a process of human personal and spiritual growth? And of course, this raises the question of what struggles may be necessary and of constructive value and which may constitute unnecessary detours in life and are best avoided completely.

At the very least, it is clear that for anyone only interested in so-called recreational use or getting high, the major psychedelic substances are poor choices. As repeatedly affirmed, these molecules do indeed appear to be intrinsically sacred, can trigger unanticipated experiences, and can be incredibly powerful. They may lead one through excruciating personal pain, which, though perhaps potentially meaningful in the big picture of human development for some, also can be very disruptive at the time. In the poignant words of Huston Smith, "Ecstasy is not fun."

Some of the reports of psychedelic use outside of medical or religious contexts reflect an alarming lack of knowledge. There are young people who have taken entheogens and then wandered through shopping centers or walked aimlessly through different landscapes without any intention beyond "seeing what might happen," and sometimes without the presence of any companion to help to ensure safety. One young man took pride in watching horror films on his television set and expressed a special fondness for Alfred Hitchcock's *Psycho*. With low dosage, some people may get away with such behavior, at least on some occasions, and label their experiences as "cool." Eventually, however, if they persist, the seriousness of their misuse of these intrinsically sacred substances is likely to become apparent to themselves as well as others. Confrontation of fears is always in order, but there is ample grist for the mill within each of us and there is no need to supplement it with potentially distracting or disturbing stimuli from the environment or from the fantasies of other people.

The saying "it's not what happens to you but how you respond to it that matters" is exceptionally true during psychedelic sessions. As noted in the earlier chapters, the safe and productive exploration of consciousness demands a high degree of trust, courage, openness, and interpersonal grounding. If one seeks control or tries to evade emerging experiences, anxiety will build and paranoid thought processes will often occur. Paranoid people can misinterpret environmental cues and act in ways that they would view as reckless or simply stupid when their normal faculties of good judgment are functioning.

The presence of an alert and knowledgeable companion or guide is of critical importance in ensuring safety. Genuine hallucinations, though extremely rare, sometimes do occur and, however briefly, seriously impair reality testing. I recall a man in our study of LSD-assisted therapy for narcotic addiction at the Maryland Psychiatric Research Center who, when sitting up on the couch during his psychedelic session, suddenly stared wide-eyed at the vacant black leather chair opposite him. Then, suddenly, he darted for the door, intending to yank it open, run down the hallway, and sprint out of the building. As if in a football game, I tackled him at the door and held him tightly. Panicking, he pointed to the chair and informed me that we had to quickly escape from the coiled cobra in the black chair that was threatening him. Firmly, I continued to hold him and directed him to look directly into the eyes of the cobra. As he did so, he burst into tears as he experienced the cobra transforming into his mother. His body relaxed as he tumbled through emotions that he attributed to her constricting influence on his life.

This became a pivotal therapeutic experience for him and in time he came to explore even deeper meanings of the cobra, relating it to the rising of his own spiritual energy, called *kundalini shakti* in Eastern meditative disciplines. Had this man been alone or without competent supportive companions, not only would he have missed a valuable therapeutic opportunity, but while running away with impaired judgment he could have injured himself or others. As with the nocturnal nightmares most of us can recall, when one runs away from psychological conflicts the threatening specter grows bigger and one feels weaker, smaller, and increasingly anxious, often awakening in a cold sweat; when the frightening image is courageously approached and confronted, one grows stronger and insights awaken.

As has been repeatedly stated, one's intention during the action of an entheogen is of critical significance. If one genuinely seeks personal and spiritual growth, one is also motivated to confront material that may initially appear frightening or dark. We encourage an intention to "follow the arc" of the entheogenic reaction regardless of any anxieties encountered, akin to trusting the arc of an Australian boomerang that, when thrown, circles widely but returns dependably to its point of origin. With practice, one can even arrive at a point of welcoming the appearance of a dragon or similar symbolic manifestation and, like a skilled athlete, enjoy the challenge of "looking him directly in the eye" and the adventure of tumbling through whatever emotions and insights may occur during the subsequent confrontation. In illustration of this principle within consciousness, a man under the influence of ayahuasca described a visionary sequence of going deeper and deeper into the earth, moving through various dark tunnels, past crypts, roots, spider webs, and slithering insects until, somewhere in the despicable depths, he finally arrived at an ancient door. He grasped the handle, opened the door, and discovered himself at the top of a mountain with warm sunlight and blue sky above him. The mind often works like that. A helpful mantram to silently repeat during psychedelic sessions is "in and through."

In preparing volunteers for psychedelic sessions, we sometimes suggest a fantasy of opening the door to the "basement of one's life" and announcing, "I'm coming down!" One then descends with firm footsteps, carrying a bright searchlight. Intentionally, one seeks out the darkest corners one can find in the basement and shines the light into them. Sometimes this process can continue by opening a trapdoor in the basement floor and penetrating still more deeply. When this process is grounded in the relationship with the companion or guide, there is nothing that cannot be "seen for what it is." One may affirm an inherent right to know what is going on within one's own mind. Ultimately this intention leads to the resolution of anything within that has potential to engender anxiety and an awareness that it is safe to relax and genuinely to be at peace. With this intention and interpersonal grounding during the action of a psychedelic substance, it is common to hear the report, "There is nothing to fear."

The safety record during the past fifteen years of research at Johns Hopkins has been consistently positive. Though some people have indeed experienced difficult episodes of anxiety during their psychedelic sessions, sufficient new insights and perspectives have also emerged so that in retrospect the experiences are viewed as constructive and meaningful. To my knowledge, no person to date who has completed participation in a study has reported regret at having volunteered or any adverse impact on his or her personal or spiritual life.

This situation may well be attributed to the careful medical and psychological screening that all volunteers undergo, and also to the interpersonal climate in the research unit. Volunteers are welcomed as valued participants and colleagues on an important frontier of knowledge rather than labeled as "patients" or "experimental subjects." A similar therapeutic climate and safety record prevailed in earlier research at the Spring Grove Hospital and Maryland Psychiatric Research Center and at many, if not most, other sites, past and present, where studies with entheogens and normal volunteers or persons seeking psychotherapeutic treatment have been conducted.

Further, once a person is accepted into a study and signs an informed consent document, he or she usually participates in a minimum of eight hours of relationship-building time with the guide or therapist who will be present during the period of entheogen action. Typically during this period, spread over at least one or often two or three weeks, one's life history is shared in confidence, including important relationships, career developments, religious or nonreligious history and present orientation, travel experiences, and any unique traumas or accomplishments that have occurred thus far in life.

On the day before the entheogen session is scheduled, the guide surveys the varieties of experiences that could occur with the participant, insofar as words can communicate, thereby offering the best wisdom we have available on the art of maximizing opportunities for safety and benefit. This always is done in person to provide opportunities for discussion and interaction, thereby further solidifying the relationship.

Listening to a generic video on how best to respond during the action of an entheogen would not be the same. Also, each volunteer becomes familiar with the room in which the entheogen will be administered, lying on a couch, listening to music with sleepshade and headphones, often also exploring his or her own mental imagery, akin to a waking dream without the assistance of an entheogen. This becomes a "dress rehearsal" for the upcoming psychedelic session.

Another important factor in ensuring safety is the provision of trained and skilled guides. Although ideally all would have had training experiences themselves that included personally receiving entheogens, this is not always possible in the current legal-political climate in the United States and in many other countries. At a minimum, all guides in the Hopkins studies have personal experience in meditative techniques and are familiar with some alternative forms of consciousness. They have also worked in an apprentice relationship with more experienced guides, are emotionally stable and centered, and are cognitively open to the potential value of nonordinary states of awareness. Thus, they are not inclined to be fearful of unusual speech or other atypical behavior. Were a guide to become tense or worried that a person is "going crazy" and might "get out of control," that anxiety easily could become contagious, disruptive, and counterproductive.

Part of a new guide's orientation at Johns Hopkins entails becoming familiar with the supportive music used in a particular research study and the rationale for its selection. We have learned that in high-dose sessions, especially during the onset and intense period of entheogen effects, the supportive structure of the music is more important than either the guide's or the volunteer's personal musical preferences. In states of ego transcendence, the everyday self as the perceiver of music may no longer exist, having entered into a unitive awareness that is claimed to be quite independent of whatever sonic frequencies are coming into the ears through the headphones or loudspeakers. As the ego approaches its dissolution and when it begins to be reconstituted, however, the nonverbal structure of the music may provide significant support. Thus, sensitivity to the therapeutic potential of carefully selected music may be an important factor in enhancing psychological safety.

One playlist that has been carefully developed through trial and error and has been found to work well with many different people over time is included at the end of this book. It includes a significant amount of classical music, symphonic and choral, as well as some Hindu chant, in the intense portions of the session and lighter selections near the return to everyday reality at the end of the day. We discovered in early research in the 1960s, notably with some alcoholics who had never appreciated classical music, that Brahms symphonies and similar works resonated deeply within them and proved highly effective in providing nonverbal structure and support. Many of those people not only discovered an appreciation of classical music within themselves, but went out and purchased records, tapes, or compact disks to facilitate the continuing integration of their experiences and for future enjoyment. It may be noted that, as consciousness is returning to ordinary awareness after intense experiences of a mystical, visionary, or psychodynamic nature, most any style of music can be explored with delight. At this time, one's personal favorite selections may be enjoyed with fresh appreciation.

Still another important consideration in ensuring psychological safety is the provision of continuing opportunities for the integration of the psychological or spiritual content that was experienced during the action of the entheogen. In most research studies, participants who receive entheogens are encouraged to write a description of their experiences, or at least an outline or initial rough draft, on the evening of the session or early the following morning to freshly capture the essence of their insights in their own words. This helps to launch the integrative process, provides an important research document, and ensures that each volunteer has a souvenir that often remains of value in future years. With report in hand, volunteers return to the research center on the day immediately after their sessions for an appointment with their guides, initially to talk through whatever happened. The process of interpersonal sharing and discussion, including the full spectrum of thoughts, emotions, and insights, appears to solidify the benefits obtained.

Sometimes there are traumatic memories from childhood that have never been shared with anyone that need to be discussed honestly. Sometimes there are spiritual experiences beyond what the person ever conceived as being within the realm of possibility that need to be acknowledged. There are times when volunteers may be groping for words or concepts and the guides are able to normalize their experiences by articulating ways of thinking that others have found helpful or by suggesting readings from the writings of mystics from years past or of more recent explorers of the mind. Research protocols usually provide several hours for integration after a psychedelic session occurs to help to ensure safety and to continue to solidify potentially beneficial responses. Yet the process of integration for many people continues for months, years, and even decades as psychological and spiritual growth advances.

In religious contexts outside of the structures of psychopharmacological research, psychological safety is promoted by the traditions, behavioral guidelines, and interpersonal context of the spiritual community. Religious elders often fulfill the role of guides and the community as a whole provides the respectful acceptance required to integrate both psychologically painful and spiritually ecstatic experiences. In one study, Paulo Cesar Ribeiro Barbosa and his colleagues surveyed fifteen publications that had evaluated emotional, cognitive, or physical health responses reported after the acute effects of ayahuasca had subsided. While noting possible methodological biases in some studies, they concluded, "The accumulated data suggest that ayahuasca use is safe and may even be, under certain circumstances, beneficial." Two other recent small studies of the religious use of ayahuasca have similarly supported claims of fundamental safety, one by John Halpern of thirty-two members of a branch of the Santo Daime Church and one by Charles Grob of fifteen male members of the União do Vegetal. In both cases procedures of preparation and social support were provided within the community context.

LEGAL CONSIDERATIONS

In considering questions of safety and potential benefit, obviously possible legal consequences must also be weighed when people choose to use psychedelic substances outside of the scientific research projects, religious organizations, or other circumstances currently approved in a particular country. If one is fined or imprisoned, the psychological or spiritual benefits may well continue, but one's life can be adversely impacted.

As we thoughtfully recover from the hysteria of the 1960s, especially if present and future research projects continue to support the basic safety of the major entheogens when they are appropriately and responsibly used, it is reasonable to anticipate gradual changes in the drug laws of various countries and of their individual states or provinces. As with marijuana at the present time (2015), federal and state laws may contradict each other. For example, in the State of New Mexico in 2005 an appeals court ruled that growing psilocybin mushrooms for personal use could not be considered "manufacturing a controlled substance," but psilocybin still remains illegal in that state under federal law. The laws tend to be complex, sometimes with subtle differences between natural and synthetic forms and varying with the assumed intent associated with cultivation, transport, sale, or possession. There rarely appears to be a category of "responsible use"; possession alone is usually assumed to imply "abuse." Fortunately, the Internet provides fairly up-to-date information on current laws in different locales.

PART V

Onward

17

Fears of Awakening

One reliable effect of visionary and mystical states of consciousness is that they awaken us once again to more fully experience awe. Instead of taking life for granted as we perform our routines in everyday existence, suddenly the very fact that we are at all may seem like a miracle. It was the German philosopher Wilhelm Gottfried von Schelling who apparently first captured the attention of scholars by asking, "Why is there something and not nothing?" The fact that we are at all is pretty incredible when we think about it, even if most of us only have an adventure on earth that lasts a hundred years or less. The memory of my first philosophy professor, Arthur Munk at Albion College, comes to mind, who in class discussion would sometimes become very excited and animated, exclaiming, "What a wonderful question!," irrespective of whether or not anyone had any idea of what the answer might be.

In the wake of mystical consciousness, there tends to be a certain freshness of being and an openness to new perspectives on reality. Typically, there is little question that our intellects are very primitive, peering into the unknown on the edge of an incredibly vast mystery. When browsing in a German bookstore after my first glimpse of mystical consciousness as a young student, I found my attention captivated by a little book by Joseph Möller titled *Vielleicht ist alles anders* (Maybe,

Everything Is Different). I bought it for the title alone. Another title that intrigued me in those days was Alfred North Whitehead's *The Adventures of Ideas*. Ideas, even those that significantly influence civilizations and the course of history, rise and fall in the potency of their influence and sometimes morph into new forms.

Why is it that some of us in the human family apparently do not want to see more than routine existence? Is it fear of the unknown? Is the world too big and scary even to try to think about it? Is it even fear of being surprised, or being wrong, or not being in control? Might there be a gene for philosophizing or spiritual questing that only becomes expressed in some of us at certain times in life? When people have come to me for help with their fears of flying in airplanes, I have sometimes wondered if I should mention to them that we have always been flying on a little planet that spins (at the equator) at a speed of about one thousand miles per hour and that zooms around the sun every year at around sixty-seven thousand miles per hour. Much as we like to affirm our independence in everyday life, it remains true that, when we eventually find ourselves lying on our deathbeds, we all have to come to terms with an ultimate dependency on realities far greater than our egos. Why is it that I think of the title of the book by C. S. Lewis *Surprised by Joy*?

I recall the day some years ago when my wife and I decided to do something nice for her elderly aunt, Tante Wilma. Wilma's life was limited; she was a widow who lived alone in a small apartment in a suburb of Dortmund in Germany. We decided to take her by train to Amsterdam for a day. One could see trouble brewing when we picked her up, as she insisted on wearing a heavy long black coat on a hot July day. When the border police checked our passports as the train entered Holland, she became exceptionally anxious, perhaps reliving memories from World War II. Finally we arrived in Amsterdam, climbed aboard a streetcar, and made our way to the Van Gogh Museum. She complained that we had not yet seen the queen of the Netherlands and then planted herself in a chair in the entrance hall of the museum, immediately adjacent to an open archway, beyond which some of the most magnificent of Van Gogh's paintings were hanging. There she firmly sat, sulking, absolutely refusing to look around the corner, much less actually humoring or placating us by taking a few steps through the archway. When we finally returned her to her apartment late that evening, she made it clear that the day had been a terrible and most unpleasant ordeal.

Trying to view Tante Wilma with compassion, we can see her suffering from the constricted consciousness we often call depression, stubbornly living in ways that exacerbate her distress while avoiding the beauty and life that are all around her. Perhaps precisely what she feared most was joy. In DSM V, the diagnostic and statistical manual of politically sanctioned terms used by mental health providers to label patients for insurance reimbursement, the diagnosis "fear of joy" is noticeably absent.

Similarly, I recall one of the theological students with whom I was asked to sit as he experienced his first psilocybin session in Dr. Leuner's clinic. I didn't know much about the art of guiding sessions then, and should have been alerted when he turned his back to me, buried his face deep in the inner corners of the couch cushions, and remained silent and nonresponsive to my attempts to communicate with him. Finally, as the effect of the entheogen was waning, he exclaimed, "Ich habe es geschafft!" (I made it!). It turned out that during the entire session he had experienced a whirlpool that steadily attempted to draw him into a vortex leading into the depths of the ocean. Instead of affirming trust and diving into the depths, allowing the visionary waters and even his apprentice guide to support him, he had spent the entire time swimming valiantly and energetically against the current and now felt quite exhausted. At least on that day, he missed an opportunity to discover the treasures, whether insightfully painful or joyful, that might have awaited him in the depths of his mind. Psychologically, we would call his behavior "resistance" and fear of relinquishing control.

A third example comes from an unforgettable morning when I visited two different cancer patients, approximately of the same age. One happened to be a woman from an exceptionally wealthy family. We prepared for her LSD session, sitting beside her swimming pool in a luxurious suburb of Baltimore, attended by servants. I recall that she apologized that her living room still had furnishings in it from the prior year since her interior decorator hadn't updated them yet. The other was a poverty-stricken woman who lived in a poorly maintained row house in Baltimore's slums. We met in her kitchen with torn linoleum on the floor and cockroaches, long since accepted as inevitable housemates, literally crawling on our bodies. Both women were confronting the same issue: the imminence of death. Perhaps due to my own limitations, two attempts to assist the wealthy woman with the help of LSD failed, and she finally died, isolated, depressed, and bitter. Death was the one thing she could not control, an awareness that triggered a response to life that can best be described as seething anger and sulking. In contrast, the woman in the slums was able to respond to the opportunity provided by the psychedelic substance with openness and gratitude and approached death with interpersonal warmth and a sense of inner peace.

There are many people, including a significant number of mental health professionals, who have come to assume that the use of psychedelic substances is intrinsically dangerous. Without comprehension of dosage, the significance of set (personality structure, preparation, and expectations) and setting (the physical and social environment), and the varieties of alternative states of awareness, they have assumed that the responses to entheogens are unpredictable and capricious. Some who have personally ingested one of the psychedelic substances have encountered frightening states of consciousness and appear to have little motivation to come to understand their inner conflicts and unpleasant experiences; others have known friends, family members, or patients who "got into trouble" and had used psychedelics and, on that basis, assume it is inadvisable for anyone to ingest them. Some psychiatrists know only the mental health casualties that appear in emergency rooms, akin to internists who have to cope with the victims of automobile accidents. They tend not to see those who value beneficial experiences, largely because use outside of prescribed medical and religious settings is currently illegal and psychiatric assistance may not be required.

The ways we are taught to perceive drugs in early childhood can still be quite pervasive and persuasive in adulthood. Regarding alcohol, though born after the cultural experiment called prohibition (1920–1933), I grew up with an active chapter of the Women's Christian Temperance Union (WCTU) in my Methodist church. In a rather simplistic manner, I was taught that if no one consumed alcohol, there would be no alcoholism. As I grew older and began to question authority a bit more, I realized that the teaching was similar to saying that if no one drove an automobile, there would be no car accidents. In this little iron mining community called Negaunee, there were twenty-two taverns along the main downtown street, which was only two blocks long. I now appreciate that those taverns must have met some of the social needs of many residents, most of whom toiled in rather dismal underground tunnels during long daytime hours.

My own home, however, was alcohol-free, except occasionally for a few drops of brandy in the Christmas fruitcake. When good old Mrs. Baldasari presented my father, the high school principal, with a bottle of her homemade wine in appreciation of his interventions with her son, the bottle sat in the cabinet under our kitchen sink for almost a year. Finally, as a self-righteous kid in junior high school, the day came when I poured the evil substance down the drain to the continuing consternation of my older brother over sixty years later. Alcohol had an emotional charge for me then, and I vividly recall a drunken man loudly knocking on our door and lewdly wanting to talk with my frightened mother. Earlier in his life, he had been a promising concert pianist; now, allegedly due to alcohol, he was the town shoemaker who listened to recordings made of his performances on stages in Chicago years ago while he stitched soles and hammered heels. I also recall, when hiking in the uncharted wilderness, coming upon a long-abandoned copper kettle and condensing coil almost completely covered by vines and underbrush deep in the woods where a couple decades earlier someone had illegally built a still and manufactured taboo moonshine. If caught, he would have been imprisoned back then. As I matured, I gradually became more tolerant of alcohol, but still did not drink my first beer until I literally left the shores of the United States on a German ship, bound for Europe. Those early Sunday school lessons on "the evils of alcohol" had deeply penetrated my mind. I realize now that those who grew up in homes with well-stocked bars and parents who not only enjoyed drinks before, during, and after dinner but considered offering alcohol integral to polite and gracious hospitality viewed the substance from a totally different perspective.

During the past few decades, I've come to enjoy an occasional glass of wine with a fine meal or a bottle of beer with Maryland crabs, but have still never developed a personal taste for cocktails and casual social drinking. I have learned to appreciate that attitudes change slowly with education and life experiences. I remain concerned about alcohol abuse, have witnessed friends dying from cirrhosis of the liver, and have empathized with many private patients, research volunteers, and their family members while attempting to treat people suffering from addiction to alcohol. Yet I would not vote for the renewed prohibition of alcohol and believe that many people can responsibly integrate the substance into their diets and social lives. In moderation, alcohol may provide pleasant taste sensations, some health benefits, and feelings of enhanced relaxation and social camaraderie. Unlike psychedelic substances, it rarely if ever provides insights or knowledge relevant to personal and spiritual growth. Also, unlike psychedelic substances, alcohol is physically addictive and causes physiological damage.

Now if psychedelic sacraments have the capacity to awaken us to genuinely spiritual knowledge, why would any government fear them, declare them illegal, and go so far as to threaten imprisonment of people who may find certain species of mushrooms growing in their yards? Why is it that current federal regulations in the United States require that the psilocybin approved for research use be kept in a locked safe, bolted to the ground if the safe weighs less than 750 pounds, in a secure facility? It is only an intrinsically sacred substance that Indians have calmly used in their religious rituals for at least three thousand years, if not significantly longer; it is not a radioactive isotope.

Yet at this point in American history, as observed earlier, research with these compounds requires clearance from two federal agencies: the Food and Drug Administration (FDA) and the Drug Enforcement Administration (DEA), plus careful approval by the local Institutional Review Board (IRB) that oversees projects of research, protecting human subjects by weighing risk-benefit ratios, examining completeness of informed consent documents, and confirming the scientific integrity of the research designs. As clearly outlined in a recent article, published in *Nature Reviews* by three experts in psychopharmacology, David Nutt, Leslie King, and David Nichols, the current governmental controls and legal strictures have seriously impeded progress in scientific research with psychedelic compounds internationally. Until very recently, it appeared that government funding would only be considered for research that intended to document some adverse effect of their use; any studies of potentially positive uses seemed to be outside of the scope of governmental interest. This situation is especially mind-boggling in countries where many college students and other citizens are choosing to use psychedelics. One would hope that federal agencies with responsibility for the health of all its citizens would want to obtain all information possible about responses to different entheogens by promoting and funding scientific research; to date, unfortunately, this has rarely been the case.

Actually, the patchwork of laws and their enforcement in different parts of the world is quite fascinating. Though the growth of any of the 180 or so species of psilocybin-containing mushrooms in your backyard is generally deemed illegal in most states and provinces, in 2005 the Louisiana legislature, for example, went so far as to forbid the growing of two species of morning glories (*Ipomea violacea* and *Rivea corymbosa*), unless used "strictly for aesthetic, landscaping or decorative purposes." There are at least three varieties of morning glories purported to produce seeds that have psychoactive effects, because they contain lysergic acid amide (LSA), a substance similar to LSD that merits additional scientific investigation. One cannot help but wonder about the origin of the names of these species, since they are known as Heavenly Blue, Pearly Gates, and Flying Saucers. Called "ololiuqui," a white species that botanists call *Turbina* (or *Rivea*) *corymbosa* have been used by Indians in Central America in their religious ceremonies for at least two hundred years, sometimes along with psilocybin-containing mushrooms.

Morning glory seeds, especially those that may have been sprayed with other chemicals in seed packets, are probably not ideal entheogenic substances and, like many natural plant entheogens, contain numerous compounds, some of which may contribute to nausea or other adverse effects. The same legislation in Louisiana specified thirty-eight other plants and fungi, including the *Banisteriopsis caapi* vine, which, though not even containing an entheogen, is used in the preparation of the sacramental ayahuasca drink. The legislation also specified the *Psilocybe* genus of mushrooms and the bright red mushroom with white spots known as *Amanita muscaria* that appears to have a long history and, risky as its use may be by uninformed persons, may have been a contributing factor in the origins of Judeo-Christian religions according to John Allegro. It appears that governments, for better or worse, have really been engaged in a "plant war." Some would also call it a war within consciousness and might view it as the evolutionary birth pangs of increasing spiritual awareness in the human species.

Perhaps all these cautious safeguards currently in place, extreme and unnecessarily alarmist as they may appear, not to mention frustrating to qualified and dedicated researchers, are understandable as we recover from the cultural traumas of the 1960s with the clash of values surrounding the Vietnam War, race relations, the women's movement, and the sexual revolution. This cultural conflict in our history is often illustrated by the extreme stereotypes of Western students offering flowers to soldiers, chanting Hare Krishna, and saying "make love, not war" at one pole, and the equally distorted specter of industrial giants exclusively obsessed with immediate economic gains and aggressive military strategies on the other. It might help in the present climate for us to honestly acknowledge that we as a global society have indeed been traumatized, that we appear to have hysterically overreacted, and that we often still tend to be confused and ambivalent in our thinking about entheogenic substances in either plant or pharmaceutically pure forms.

Perhaps in our collective psyche, there is a desire to avoid grief and guilt that originate in the violence we have perpetuated in the world, ranging from our recent struggles to cope intelligently with tensions in Southeast Asia and the Middle East to our wars with American Indians in the colonial era. We make and implement the best decisions we can in times of crisis, but we still invariably incur guilt that is more easily denied than confronted and resolved. As Karl Jaspers expressed when the Third Reich finally collapsed and World War II came to a close in his book *Die Schuldfrage* (translated as *The Question of German Guilt*), all citizens inevitably incur guilt by failing to become informed, to monitor political trends, and to honestly express the voices of their consciences.

As many of us know, the improbable does occasionally happen. We tend to call them "incredible coincidences." In May 1943, while British and American fighter planes were dropping bombs on the city of Dortmund, a little blonde girl, seven years of age, courageously stood beside her papa at the entrance of their neighborhood bunker, watching the spectacular flares in the sky and listening to the deafening explosions. Destruction was everywhere; most everyone was traumatized. In August 1972, now a thirty-six-year-old psychiatric nurse and my wife, she found herself guiding a terminal cancer patient through a psychedelic session with dipropyltryptamine (DPT) at Sinai Hospital in Baltimore. This man, a former fighter pilot in the US Air Force, had literally sat in the bombing bay of one of those planes and in repeated attacks had released bombs over Dortmund. He was twenty years old at the time of the bombings and now, at age forty-nine, still recalled how much he enjoyed "shooting Nazis." As they held each other's hands during and after his DPT session, sharing their mutual appreciation for Beethoven and Brahms, as well as their human connection in the present, there was also shared awareness that both had been caught up in powerful currents of world events that dwarfed their individual lives. What now prevailed was acceptance and reconciliation on the threshold of one man's death in a very different period of history.

It always is fashionable in times of cultural transition to convene task forces of experts and to call for additional study and research, and such activity is always needed and welcome. At the present time an increasing number of scientists in various countries are in the process of carefully investigating the safety of the responsible use of different psychedelic substances and their findings will continue to appear in professional journals. Yet there has been a tendency to ignore the abundance of knowledge that has already been published in years past, as if the wheel needs once again to be reinvented. I hope that, if we combine past and present research, and if the safety and potential benefit of psychedelic substances continues to be supported, cultural controls can gradually be relaxed in sane and responsible ways. Their present classification in Schedule I in the United States as drugs that have "no currently accepted medical use" and have a "lack of accepted safety for use under medical supervision" is outdated and no longer accurate or appropriate. Whether or not such drugs have "a high potential for abuse" is debatable, insofar as they are nonaddictive, there was little respect for serious and knowledgeable "use" when the repressive legislation was enacted, and there are many other substances not listed in any schedule, such as alcohol, caffeine, and nicotine, that also have their own potentials for abuse. Within the next few years, it is anticipated that well-designed studies with increasingly large samples of participants will provide substantial recent data to inform intelligent decision making.

18

Entering Into a New Paradigm

All this cultural change may be seen as occurring in the context of an even larger change, often called a paradigm shift. A paradigm may be defined as the big grid of assumptions and perceptions by which the majority of people view reality. Thomas Kuhn employed the term in his book *The Structure of Scientific Revolutions*. It is a question of exactly whose "reality" has become the baseline, shared by the largest number of people in a civilization. As illustrated by the tale of the "hundredth monkey," there comes a time when a minority evolves into a majority, when a shift in consciousness occurs, and what once was considered highly improbable suddenly becomes obvious, reasonable, and accepted. "Of course," people say, "What's the big deal?" Women are bright enough to vote. Skin color has nothing to do with worth, talent, or opportunity. One genuinely can love, be responsible, and contribute to society regardless of sexual identity.

Consider the shift in paradigm that occurred when Ptolemaic astronomy gave way to the Copernican view of the universe. In Ptolemaic astronomy, the earth was flat and heavenly bodies moved in irregular paths through the skies called epicycles amid beautiful crystalline spheres. Aristotle and Pope Paul V subscribed to this view and if you said the flat earth was not the center of the universe on a test, you were informed that your answer was wrong. Many doctoral theses in those days in all probability reported detailed observations of the irregular, jagged "epicycles" that various stars traveled as they moved across the firmament. The observations, even then, may have been reasonably accurate, though today we would consider the framework in which they were interpreted primitive and in error.

Now we've pretty much adjusted to the Copernican, or heliocentric, view of the world, though we still talk about sunrises and sunsets instead of turns of a rotating earth. Contemporary astronomy stretches our imaginations farther and farther and we are now aware of countless galaxies far beyond our own Milky Way and measure distances in light years. The lobby of the Space Telescope Institute on the campus of the Johns Hopkins School of Arts and Sciences contains a large backlit mural filled with what looks like an incredible panorama of bright stars; in reality, most of the points of lights are not stars, but distant galaxies. It continues to amaze me that employees casually can walk past it with their brown-bag lunches without, at least occasionally, falling prostrate on the floor, overcome with awe and wonder.

If the intuitive insights that are reliably reported in mystical states of consciousness are indeed valid, space, time, and substance may eventually be understood in the context of yet another paradigm of reality, one quantum physicists already seem to begin to comprehend. As earlier noted, we all sort of accept that the desk at which we sit, solid as it may appear to be, is actually really made up of whirling subatomic particles. It is really energy in motion and is ultimately not the solid fibers we perceive with our eyes and our fingertips. Perhaps the same is true of our bodies.

Galileo Galilei in the early seventeenth century, as brilliantly depicted by the German playwright Bertolt Brecht, was among the first to question the Ptolemaic view of reality. Unlike the philosopher Giordano Bruno, who was burned at the stake for questioning the dominant worldview only a decade earlier, Galileo had a newly invented tool called the telescope. With this tool he could observe that the moons of Jupiter periodically disappeared as they rotated behind the planet. This observation he considered empirical evidence to support the Copernican perspective.

In Brecht's play, Galileo is depicted as being surrounded by the authorities of his day–a philosopher, a theologian, and a mathematician (authorities change!)–and he invites them to look through his telescope and see for themselves that a new fascinating and awesome paradigm of reality is emerging. However, they refuse to look and comment that, even if they did peer into the silly tube, and even if they saw what Galileo claimed, they would know it was only a hallucination. After all, the pope and Aristotle were in agreement that the earth was flat. Furthermore, telescopes were being used by rebellious youth for voyeuristic purposes, so no responsible parent would allow his or her child to have a telescope. Galileo is censored and put under house arrest; yet the vistas he experienced remained valid and would become acknowledged by future generations. It is worth noting that the paradigm shift ultimately did not even threaten theologians, but instead revealed an even more vast and magnificent universe. The crystalline spheres were beautiful, but so are distant nebulae and galaxies.

19

Movement Into the Future

Alan Watts (1915–1973), one of the first theologically trained scholars to begin to introduce people in Western cultures to Eastern religions, notably Zen Buddhism, wrote about "the taboo of knowing who you are." If we take mystical consciousness seriously and accept that it appears to be a potential state of awareness that ultimately awaits all of us, then eventually we may all have to accept that we are spiritual beings, that there is indeed "something of God within us," and that, whether we like it or not, the time is coming when we may have to put up with being unconditionally loved.

What would our world be like if more of us were awakening spiritually, if more of us were increasingly aware of both the temporal and the eternal realms in consciousness? Such awareness appears to be dawning and intensifying in the minds of many people, as evidenced by the expanding interest in yoga and meditative disciplines, by curiosity about and tolerance for the perspectives of different world religions, as well as in expanding respect for the therapeutic, educational, and sacramental use of psychedelic substances.

In our current evolution, fueled by the constructive use of technology, increasing international travel, and the Internet, diversity and intercultural communication are becoming increasingly valued. With fresh

fresh creativity and growing understanding of other societies and religious perspectives, perhaps more of our tensions can actually be resolved by respectful dialogues in the chambers of the United Nations and between individual countries rather than on physical battlefields. Is there really anything immoral or demented about loving instead of making war? The love intuited in mystical states is not wimpy and naïve; it tends to be reported as intelligent, wise, and incredibly powerful. It can be expressed in reaching out to other cultures with a disciplined determination to master their histories, their social and economic situations, and their religions and their languages, and to enter into intercultural dialogues respectfully, humbly, and patiently.

One could suggest that our wars and conflicts are integral parts of the unfolding divine drama, simply a manifestation of the dance of Shiva. Clashing, dissonant chord progressions, after all, have their reason for being and are incorporated into the magnificence of a symphony; an endlessly sustained C-major chord would get pretty boring. Yet, within time and the evolution of our species, it appears that we could well be moving toward a more peaceful world utopia of some kind. If the intuitions of mystics are valid and consciousness continues after the deaths of physical bodies, one could even ask whether killing on battlefields is meaningful or effective, or whether there are more evolved ways of interacting with those who view the world differently than we do and who believe and act in ways we find difficult to comprehend.

If psychedelic substances, responsibly and wisely employed, are indeed going to become valued tools in understanding ourselves, our fellow human beings, and the universe in which we discover ourselves, many adjustments in our current attitudes, procedures, and laws gradually need to be made. In what ways should legal access and possession be granted? Who should be the guardians held responsible for their wise use? Should mental health professionals be the gate- keepers with psychiatrists writing prescriptions? Should religious professionals decide when one is ready to receive what has been called "the sacrament that works"? Should membership in a religion where entheogens are accepted as sacraments be required for legal access, or can freedom of religion be honored outside of affiliation with a particular church, synagogue, temple, or mosque? Can the man on the street be adequately educated or held responsible to obtain the requisite knowledge in order to make his or her own decisions about whether and how and when to use psychedelics? We allow this with alcohol, nicotine, caffeine, and increasingly marijuana, knowing that some will use the substances inappropriately and abusively while many will use them responsibly. How can the purity, accurate labeling, and proper dosage of psychedelic substances best be ensured so that the probability of safety and effectiveness can be maximized? These are all important issues for us to explore, and the time is now.

Personally, I envision continuing research projects of many kinds that are designed to investigate the promise of responsibly integrating psychedelic substances into our culture. In the immediate future, they will require the approval and oversight of governmental agencies and Institutional Review Boards. Such studies could focus not only on potential medical applications, but, as outlined in this book, also on educational and religious uses. Social scientists have the skills to monitor and measure the beneficial or detrimental effects discovered by such studies.

Many of these studies could proceed under the aegises of universities and research institutions. Others could occur in experimental retreat centers, some located in scenic natural settings, where people who desire a legal psychedelic experience could apply, receive medical screening and counsel, have access to pure substances in proper dosage, receive competent preparation, guidance, and support as needed during the periods of alternate states of consciousness, and obtain initial integrative assistance in individual and group contexts. Such centers, in the countries that would sponsor and support them, would be staffed by interdisciplinary professionals, both medical and religious. They would also include teams of social scientists well trained in the procedures of research. I hope to live long enough, if not to participate as a staff member at such a center, at least to have the honor of visiting one. As an American citizen, I would be especially proud if one of the first centers was successfully established in my own country.

Epilogue

A Concise Report of Insights from the Frontier
Where Science and Spirituality Are Meeting

(Some suggestions to consider and explore)

1. In case you had any doubts, God (or whatever your favorite noun for ultimate reality may be) is.
2. God awaits and embraces us both as Ground of Being (Celestial Buddha Fields, Pure Land, The Void that contains all Reality, The Ground Luminosity of Pure Awareness) and as Personal Deity (Lord Jehovah, Lord Jesus, Lord Krishna, Lord Buddha).
3. There are heavens and hells within each of us and they are magnificently designed.
4. The ultimate nature of matter and mind (if you take the mystics seriously) appears to be an ontological source or force of energy called love.
5. Consciousness, whether we like it or not, appears to be indestructible.
6. We are really more than we know of ourselves and can experience visionary content that does not arise from our personal developmental histories.
7. God moves in mysterious ways. When we trust and act in the world, a meaningful process unfolds within us. Each of us is still being created and crafted as a work of art.

8. There is truth in Myth.
9. True humility is awe before the unspeakable greatness of Being.
10. Beauty may be in and through the eye of the Beholder, but it can be Absolute and incredibly magnificent.
11. We are all interconnected with one another, and perhaps with all that is; the Unity of Humankind, Gaia, and the Net of Indra are very real.
12. The yearnings to know and understand truth expressed in science and philosophy are themselves encompassed within the temporal rivers that flow into the eternal ocean.
13. What is *is*–stretching beyond our most favorite words and concepts.

SELECTED BIBLIOGRAPHY

ARTICLES

Barbosa, Paulo Cesar Ribeiro, Suely Mizumoto, Michael P. Bogenschutz, and Rick J. Strassman. 2012. "Health Status of Ayahuasca Users." *Drug Testing and Analysis* 4 (7–8): 601–609.

Barker, Steven A., Jimo Borjigin, Izabela Lomnicka, Rick Strassman. 2013. "Dimethyltryptamine Hallucinogens, Their Precursors, and Major Metabolites in Rat Pineal Gland Microdialysate." *Biomedical Chromatography* 27 (12): 1690–1700.

Bogenschutz, Michael P. 2013. "Studying the Effects of Classic Hallucinogens in the Treatment of Alcoholism: Rationale, Methodology and Current Research with Psilocybin." *Current Drug Abuse Reviews* 6 (1): 17–29.

Bogenschutz, Michael P., Alyssa A. Forcehimes, Jessica A. Pommy, Claire E. Wilcox, P.C.R. Barbosa, and Rick J. Strassman. 2015. "Psilocybin-Assisted Treatment for Alcohol Dependence: A Proof-of-Concept Study." *Journal of Psychopharmacology* 29 (3): 289–299.

Carhart-Harris, Robin, Mendel Kaelen, and David Nutt. 2014. "How Do Hallucinogens Work on the Brain?" *Psychologist* 27 (9): 662–665.

Dishotsky, Norman I., William D. Loughman, Robert E. Mogar, and Wendell R. Lipscomb. 1971. "LSD and Genetic Damage." *Science* 172 (3982): 431–440.

Garcia-Romeu, Albert, Roland R. Griffiths, Matthew W. Johnson. 2015. "Psilocybin-Occasioned Mystical Experiences in the Treatment of Tobacco Addiction." *Current Drug Abuse Reviews* 7 (3).

Gasser, Peter, Dominique Holstein, Yvonne Michel, Rick Doblin, Berra Yazar-Klosinski, Torsten Passie, and Rudolf Brenneisen. 2014. "Safety and Efficacy of Lysergic Acid Diethylamide-Assisted Psychotherapy for Anxiety Associated with Life-Threatening Diseases." *Journal of Nervous and Mental Disease* 202 (7): 513–520.

Gasser, Peter, Katharina Kirchner, and Torsten Passie. 2014. "LSD-Assisted Psychotherapy for Anxiety Associated with a Life-Threatening Disease: A Qualitative Study of Acute and Sustained Subjective Effects." *Journal of Psychopharmacology* 29 (1): 57–68.

Griffiths, Roland R., Matthew W. Johnson, William A. Richards, Brian D. Richards, Una D. McCann, and Robert Jesse. 2011. "Psilocybin Occasioned Mystical-Type Experiences: Immediate and Persisting Dose-Related Effects." *Psychopharmacology* 218 (4): 649–665.

Griffiths, Roland R., William A. Richards, Matthew W. Johnson, Una D. McCann, and Robert Jesse. 2008. "Mystical-Type Experiences Occasioned by Psilocybin Mediate the Attribution of Personal Meaning and Spiritual Significance 14 Months Later." *Journal of Psychopharmacology* 22 (6): 621–632.

Griffiths, Roland R., William A. Richards, Una McCann, and Robert Jesse. 2006. "Psilocybin Can Occasion Mystical-Type Experiences Having Substantial and Sustained Personal Meaning and Spiritual Significance." *Psychopharmacology* 187 (3): 268–283.

Grob, Charles S., Alicia L. Danforth, Gurpreet S. Chopra, Marycie Hagerty, Charles R. McKay, Adam L. Halberstadt, and George R. Greer. 2011. "Pilot Study of Psilocybin Treatment for Anxiety in Patients with Advanced-Stage Cancer." *Archives of General Psychiatry* 68 (1): 71–78.

Grob, Charles S., Dennis J. McKenna, James C. Callaway, Glacus S. Brito, Edison S. Neves, Guilherme Oberlaender, Oswaldo L. Saide, Elizeu Labigalini, Christine Tacla, Claudio T. Miranda, Rick J. Strassman, and Kyle B. Boone. 1996. "Human Psychopharmacology of Hoasca, a Plant Hallucinogen Used in Ritual Context in Brazil." *Journal of Nervous and Mental Disease* 184 (2): 86–94.

Halpern, John H., Andrea R. Sherwood, Torsten Passie, Kimberly C. Blackwell, and A. James Ruttenber. 2008. "Evidence of Health and Safety in American Members of a Religion Who Use a Hallucinogenic Sacrament." *Medical Science Monitor* 14 (8): SR15–22.

Hendricks, Peter S., C. Brendan Clark, Matthew W. Johnson, Kevin R. Fontaine, and Karen L. Cropsey. 2014. "Hallucinogen Use Predicts Reduced Recidivism Among Substance-Involved Offenders Under Community Corrections Supervision." *Journal of Psychopharmacology* 28 (1): 62–66.

Hoffman, Albert. 1997. "The Message of the Elusinian Mysteries for Today's World." In *Entheogens and the Future of Religion*, edited by Robert Forte, 31–40. San Francisco: Council on Spiritual Practices.

Hood, Ralph W. 2006. "The Common Core Thesis in the Study of Mysticism." In *Where God and Science Meet*, edited by P. McNamara, 3:119–38. Westport, Conn.: Praeger.

Hood, Ralph W., Nima Ghorbani, P. J. Watson, Ahad Framarz Ghramaleki, Mark N. Bing, H. Kristi Davison, Ronald J. Morris, and W. Paul Williamson. 2001. "Dimensions of the Mysticism Scale: Confirming the Three-Factor Structure in the United States and Iran." *Journal for the Scientific Study of Religion* 40 (4): 691–705.

Johnson, Matthew W., Albert Garcia-Romeau, Mary P. Cosimano, and Roland R. Griffiths. 2014. "Pilot Study of the 5-HT2AR Agonist Psilocybin in the Treatment of Tobacco Addiction." *Journal of Psychopharmacology* 28 (11): 983–992.

Johnson, Matthew W., William A. Richards, and Roland R. Griffiths. 2008. "Human Hallucinogen Research: Guidelines for Safety." *Journal of Psychopharmacology* 22 (6): 603–619.

Katz, Steven T. 1978. "Language, Epistemology and Mysticism." In *Mysticism and Philosophical Analysis*, edited by Steven Katz, 22–74. Oxford: Oxford University Press.

Kraehenmann, Rainer, Katrin H. Preller, Milan Scheidegger, Thomas Pokorny, Oliver G. Bosch, Eric Seifritz, and Franz X. Vollenweider. 2014. "Psilocybin-Induced Decrease in Amygdala Reactivity Correlates with Enhanced Positive Mood in Healthy Volunteers." *Biological Psychiatry*.

Krebs, Teri S., and Pål-Orjan Johansen. 2013. "Psychedelics and Mental Health: A Population Study." *PLOS ONE* 8 (8): 10.1371/journal.pone.0063972.

Leary, Timothy. 1964. "The Religious Experience: Its Production and Interpretation." *Psychedelic Review* 1 (3): 324–346.

Leary, Timothy, George H. Litwin, and Ralph Metzner. 1963. "Reactions to Psilocybin Administered in a Supportive Environment." *Journal of Nervous and Mental Disease* 137 (6): 561–573.

MacLean, Katherine A., Matthew W. Johnson, and Roland R. Griffiths. 2011. "Mystical Experiences Occasioned by the Hallucinogen Psilocybin Lead to Increases in the Personality Domain of Openness." *Journal of Psychopharmacology* 25 (11): 1453–1461.

Moreno, Francisco A., Christopher B. Wiegand, E. K. Taitano, and Pedro L. Delgado. 2006. "Safety, Tolerability and Efficacy of Psilocybin in 9 Patients with Obsessive-Compulsive Disorder." *Journal of Clinical Psychiatry* 67 (11): 1735–1740.

Nutt, David J., Leslie A. King, and David E. Nichols. 2013. "Effects of Schedule I Drug Laws on Neuroscience Research and Treatment Innovation." *Nature Reviews: Neuroscience* 14:577–585.

Pahnke, Walter N., and William A. Richards. 1966. "Implications of LSD and Experimental Mysticism." *Journal of Religion and Health* 5:175–208.

Pollan, Michael. 2015. "The Trip Treatment." *New Yorker*, February 9, 36–47.

Richards, William A. 2014. "Here and Now: Discovering the Sacred with Entheogens." *Zygon: Journal of Religion and Science* 49 (3): 652–665.

Roberts, Thomas B. 2014. "From the 500-Year Blizzard of Words to Personal Sacred Experiences–the New Religious Era." In *Seeking the Sacred with Psychoactive*

Substances: Chemical Paths to Spirituality and to God, edited by J. Harold Ellens, 1:1–22. Santa Barbara: Praeger/ABC-CLIO.

Sewell, R. Andrew, John H. Halpern, and Harrison G. Pope, Jr. 2006. "Response of Cluster Headache to Psilocybin and LSD." *Neurology* 66 (12): 1920–1922.

Tjio, Joe-Hin, Walter N. Pahnke, and Albert A. Kurland. 1969. "LSD and Chromosomes: A Controlled Experiment." *Journal of the American Medical Association (JAMA)* 210 (5): 849–856.

Tupper, Kenneth W. 2002. "Entheogens and Existential Intelligence: The Use of Plant Teachers as Cognitive Tools." *Canadian Journal of Education* 27 (4): 499–516.

—. 2003. Entheogens and Education: Exploring the Potential of Psychoactives as Educational Tools." *Journal of Drug Education and Awareness* 1 (2): 145–161.

Yensen, Richard, and Donna Dryer. 1995. "Thirty Years of Psychedelic Research: The Spring Grove Experiment and Its Sequels." In *Worlds of Consciousness: Proceedings of 1094 Conference*, edited by Adolf Dittrich, Albert Hofmann, and Hanscarl Leuner, 5:141–176. Göttingen: Verlag für Wissenschaft und Bildung.

BOOKS

Allegro, John M. 1970. *The Sacred Mushroom and the Cross: A Study of the Nature and Origins of Christianity Within the Fertility Cults of the Ancient Near East.* Garden City, N.Y.: Doubleday.

Barnard, G. William. 2011. *Living Consciousness: The Metaphysical Vision of Henri Bergson.* Albany: State University of New York Press.

Bonny, Helen L., with Louis M. Savary. 2005 [1973]. *Music and Your Mind: Listening with New Consciousness.* New Braunfels, Tex.: Barcelona Publishers.

Brecht, Bertolt. 1966. *Galileo.* Translated by Charles Laughton. New York: Grove.

Brunton, Paul. 1935. *A Search in Secret India.* New York: Dutton.

Bugental, James F. 1978. *Psychotherapy and Process.* New York: McGraw-Hill.

Campbell, Joseph. 2008 [1949]. *The Hero with a Thousand Faces.* 2nd ed. San Francisco: New World Library.

Capra, Fritjof. 2000 [1975]. *The Tao of Physics: An Exploration of the Parallels Between Modern Physics and Eastern Mysticism.* Boston: Shambhala.

Clark, Walter H. 1969. *Chemical Ecstasy.* New York: Sheed and Ward.

Cohen, Sidney. 1964. *The Beyond Within: The LSD Story.* New York: Atheneum.

Eck, Diana L. 1993. *Encountering God: A Spiritual Journey from Bozeman to Banaras.* Boston: Beacon.

Ellens, J. Harold, ed. 2014. *Seeking the Sacred with Psychoactive Substances: Chemical Paths to Spirituality and to God.* Vols. 1–2. Santa Barbara: Praeger/ABC-CLIO.

Ellens, Harold, and Thomas B. Roberts. 2015. *The Psychedelic Policy Quagmire: Health, Law, Freedom, and Society.* Westport, Conn.: Praeger/ABC-CLIO.

Fadiman, James. 2011. *The Psychedelic Explorer's Guide: Safe, Therapeutic and Sacred Journeys.* Rochester: Park Street Press.

Forman, Robert K. C., ed. 1990. *The Problem of Pure Consciousness: Mysticism and Philosophy.* New York: Oxford University Press.

Fox, Matthew. 1983. *Original Blessing: A Primer in Creation Spirituality.* Santa Fe: Bear.

Goldsmith, Neal M. 2010. *Psychedelic Healing: The Promise of Entheogens for Psychotherapy and Spiritual Development.* Rochester: Healing Arts Press.

Goldstein, Joseph, and Jack Kornfield. 1987. *Seeking the Heart of Wisdom: The Path of Insight Meditation.* Boston: Shambhala.

Grof, Stanislav. 1975. *Realms of the Human Unconscious: Observations from LSD Research.* New York: Viking.

—. 2000. *Psychology of the Future: Lessons from Modern Consciousness Research.* Albany: State University of New York Press.

—. 2005. *When the Impossible Happens: Adventures in Nonordinary Reality.* Louisville, Colo.: Sounds True.

—. 2006. *The Ultimate Journey: Consciousness and the Mystery of Death.* Ben Lomand, Calif.: Multidisciplinary Association of Psychedelic Studies.

—. 2010. *Holotropic Breathwork: A New Approach to Self-Exploration and Therapy.* Albany: State University of New York Press.

Gyatso, Tenzin (the 14th Dalai Lama). 2005. *The Universe in a Single Atom: The Convergence of Science and Spirituality.* New York: Morgan Road.

Heigl, Peter. 1980. *Mystik und Drogen-Mystik: Ein kritischer Vergleich.* Düsseldorf: Patmos.

Hesse, Herman. 1956. *Journey to the East.* Translated by Hilda Rosner. New York: Farrar, Straus and Giroux.

Hill, Scott J. 2013. *Confrontation with the Unconscious: Jungian Depth Psychology and Psychedelic Experience.* London: Muswell Hill Press.

Hofmann, Albert. 2009 [1983]. *LSD, My Problem Child: Reflections on Sacred Drugs, Mysticism and Science.* Translated by Jonathan Ott. Sarasota: Multidisciplinary Association for Psychedelic Studies.

Holland, Julie, ed. 2001. *Ecstasy: the Complete Guide, a Comprehensive Look at the Risks and Benefits of MDMA.* Rochester, Vt.: Park Street Press, 2001.

Huxley, Aldous. 1945. *The Perennial Philosophy.* New York: Harper.

—. 1963. *The Doors of Perception* and *Heaven and Hell.* New York: Harper and Row.

—. 1999. *Moksha: Aldous Huxley's Classic Writings on Psychedelics and the Visionary Experience.* Edited by Michael Horowitz and Cynthia Palmer. Rochester: Inner Traditions/Bear.

Huxley, Laura A. 2000. *This Timeless Moment: A Personal View of Aldous Huxley.* New York: Celestial Arts.

James, William. *The Varieties of Religious Experience.* New York: Modern Library, 1902.

Jaspers, Karl. 1949. *The Perennial Scope of Philosophy.* Translated by Ralph Manheim. New York: Philosophical Library.

—. 1954. *Way to Wisdom.* Translated by R. Manheim. New Haven: Yale University Press.

Josuttis, Manfred, and Hanscarl Leuner, eds. 1972. *Religion und die Droge: Ein Symposion über religiöse Erfahrungen under Einfluß von Halluzinogenen*. Stuttgart: W. Kohlhammer.

Jungaberle, Henrik, Peter Gasser, Jan Weinhold, and Rolf Verres, eds. 2008. *Therapie mit psychoaktiven Substanzen: Praxis und Kritik der Psychotherapie mit LSD, Psilocybin und MDMA*. Bern: Huber.

Kähler, Martin. 1964. *So Called Historical Jesus and the Historic Biblical Christ*. Translated by Carl E. Braaten. Minneapolis: Augsburg Fortress, 1964.

Kelly, Edward F., E. W. Kelly, A. Crabtree, A. Gauld, M. Grosso, and B. Greyson. 2007. *Irreducible Mind: Toward a Psychology for the 21st Century*. Lanham, Md.: Rowman and Littlefield.

Khan, Hazrat Inayat. 1996. *The Mysticism of Sound and Music*. Boston: Shambhala.

Kornfield, Jack. 2008. *The Wise Heart: A Guide to the Universal Teachings of Buddhist Psychology*. New York: Bantam Dell.

Kuhn, Thomas. 2012 [1962]. *The Structure of Scientific Revolutions*. Chicago: University of Chicago Press.

Lattin, Don. 2010. *The Harvard Psychedelic Club*. New York: Harper Collins.

Leary, Timothy. 1966. *Psychedelic Prayers After the Tao te Ching*. Herhonkson, N.Y.: Poets Press.

Leary, Timothy, Ralph Metzner, and Richard Alpert. 1964. *The Psychedelic Experience: A Manual Based on the Tibetan Book of the Dead*. New Hyde Park, N.Y.: University Books.

Leneghan, Sean. 2011. *The Varieties of Ecstasy Experience: An Exploration of Person, Mind and Body in Sydney's Club Culture*. Saarbrücken: LAP Lambert.

Letcher, Andrew. 2007. *Shroom: A Cultural History of the Magic Mushroom*. New York: Harper Collins.

Leuner, Hanscarl. 1981. *Halluzinogene: Psychische Grenzzustände in Forschung und Psychotherapie*. Bern: Hans Huber.

Maslow, Abraham H. 1964. *Religions, Values and Peak Experiences*. Columbus: Ohio State University Press.

—. 1966. *The Psychology of Science: A Reconnaissance*. New York: Harper and Row.

—. 1968 [1962]. *Toward a Psychology of Being*. 2nd ed. New York: Van Nostrand Reinhold.

Masters, Robert E. L., and Jean Houston. 1966. *The Varieties of Psychedelic Experience*. New York: Dell.

McNamara, Patrick, ed. 2006. *Where God and Science Meet: The Psychology of Religious Experience*. Vol. 3. Westport, Conn.: Praeger.

Merkur, Dan. 2001. *The Psychedelic Sacrament: Mana, Meditation and Mystical Experience*. Rochester: Park Street Press.

Metzner, Ralph, ed. 1968. *The Ecstatic Adventure*. New York: Macmillan.

—. 2006 [1999]. *Sacred Vine of Spirits: Ayahuasca*. Rochester: Park Street Press.

Narby, Jeremy. 1998. *The Cosmic Serpent: DNA and the Origins of Knowledge*. New York: Tarcher.

—. 2005. *Intelligence in Nature: An Inquiry Into Knowledge.* New York: Tarcher.

Newberg, Andrew B., and Eugene G. D'Aquilli. 2001. *Why God Won't Go Away: Brain Science and the Biology of Belief.* New York: Ballantine.

Otto, Rudolf. 1958 [1932]. *The Idea of the Holy.* New York: Galaxy.

Pahnke, Walter N. "Drugs and Mysticism: An Analysis of the Relationship Between Psychedelic Drugs and Mystical Consciousness." PhD diss., Harvard University. Maps.org.

Passie, Torsten, Wilfried Belschner, and Elisabeth Petrow, eds. 2013. *Ekstasen: Kontexte- Formen-Wirkungen.* Würtzburg, Ergon.

Paul, Russill. 2004. *The Yoga of Sound: Healing and Enlightenment Through the Sacred Practice of Mantra.* Novato, Calif.: New World Library.

Pollan, Michael. 2001. *The Botany of Desire: A Plant's Eye View of the World.* New York: Random House.

Powell, Simon G. 2011. *The Psilocybin Solution.* Rochester: Inner Traditions/Bear.

—. 2012. *Darwin's Unfinished Business: The Self-Organizing Intelligence of Nature.* Rochester: Park Street Press.

—. 2015. *Magic Mushroom Explorer, Psilocybin and the Awakening Earth.* Rochester: Park Street Press.

Roberts, Thomas B., ed. 2006. *Psychedelic Horizons.* Exeter: Imprint Academic.

—. 2012 [2001]. *Spiritual Growth with Entheogens: Psychoactive Sacraments and Human Transformation.* Rochester: Park Street Press.

—. 2013. *The Psychedelic Future of the Mind: How Entheogens Are Enhancing Cognition, Boosting Intelligence, and Raising Values.* Rochester: Park Street Press.

Ruck, Carl A. P. 2006. *Sacred Mushrooms of the Goddess: Secrets of Eleusis.* Berkeley: Ronin.

Sessa, Ben. 2012. *The Psychedelic Renaissance: Reassessing the Role of Psychedelic Drugs in 21st Century Psychiatry and Society.* London: Muswell Hill Press.

Shannon, Benny. 2010. *The Antipodes of the Mind: Charting the Phenomenology of the Ayahuasca Experience.* London: Oxford University Press.

Shroder, Tom. 2014. *Acid Test: LSD, Ecstasy, and the Power to Heal.* New York: Blue Rider.

Shulgin, Alexander, and Ann Shulgin. 1991. *PIHKAL: A Chemical Love Story.* Berkeley: Transform.

—. 1997. *TIHKAL: The Continuation.* Berkeley: Transform.

Sinnott, Edmund W. 1957. *Matter, Mind and Man.* New York: Harper/Atheneum.

Smith, Huston. 1976. *Forgotten Truth: The Primordial Tradition.* New York: Harper and Row.

—. 1989 [1982]. *Beyond the Post-Modern Mind.* Wheaton, Ill.: Theosophical Publishing.

—. 2000. *Cleansing the Doors of Perception: The Religious Significance of Entheogenic Plants and Chemicals.* New York: Tarcher/Putnam.

—. 2001. *Why Religion Matters: The Fate of the Human Spirit in an Age of Disbelief.* New York: HarperSanFrancisco/Harper Collins.

Smith, Huston, with Jeffrey Paine. 2009. *Tales of Wonder: Adventures Chasing the Divine*. New York: HarperOne, 2009.

Smith, Huston, and R. Snake. 1996. *One Nation Under God: The Triumph of the Native American Church*. Santa Fe: Clear Light.

Stace, Walter T. 1960. *Mysticism and Philosophy*. Philadelphia: J. B. Lippincott.

Stamets, Paul. 1996. *Psilocybin Mushrooms of the World: An Identification Guide*. Berkeley: Ten Speed.

—. 2005. *Mycelium Running: How Mushrooms Can Help Save the World*. Berkeley: Ten Speed.

Stevenson, Ian. 1980 [1974]. *Twenty Cases Suggestive of Reincarnation*. Charlottesville: University of Virginia Press.

Strassman, Rick. 2001. *DMT: The Spirit Molecule*. Rochester: Park Street Press.

—. 2014. *DMT and the Soul of Prophecy: A New Science of Spiritual Revelation in the Hebrew Bible*. Rochester: Park Street Press.

Strassman, Rick, Slawek Wojtowicz, Luis Eduardo Luna, and Ede Frecska. 2008. *Inner Paths to Outer Space: Journeys to Alien Worlds Through Psychedelics and Other Spiritual Technologies*. Rochester: Park Street Press.

Teasdale, Wayne. 1999. *The Mystic Heart*. Novato, Calif.: New World Library.

Teilhard de Chardin, Pierre. 1961. *Hymn of the Universe*. New York: Harper.

—. 1965 [1959]. *The Phenomenon of Man*. New York: Harper.

Tillich, Paul. 1952. *The Courage to Be*. New Haven: Yale University Press.

—. 1955. *Biblical Religion and the Search for Ultimate Realty*. Chicago: University of Chicago Press.

—. 1966. *The Future of Religions*. Edited by Jerald C. Brauer. New York: Harper and Row.

Wasson, Robert Gordon, Albert Hofmann, and Carl A. P. Ruck. 1998 [1978]. *The Road to Eleusis: Unveiling the Secret of the Mysteries*. Los Angeles: William Dailey Rare Books.

Wasson, Robert Gordon, Stella Kramrisch, Jonathan Ott, and Carl A. P. Ruck. 1986. *Persephone's Quest: Entheogens and the Origins of Religion*. New Haven: Yale University Press.

Watts, Alan. 1962. *The Joyous Cosmology*. New York: Pantheon.

DOCUMENTARY FILMS

Aya Awakenings: A Journey of Shamanic Discovery. 2013. Dir. Rak Razam, Icaro. www.aya-awakenings.com/watch.

Dirty Pictures. 2010. Dir. Etienne Sauret. Turn of the Century Pictures/Isis Films. www.dirtypicturesthefilm.com.

DMT: The Spirit Molecule. 2010. Dir. Mitch Schultz. Spectral Alchemy Productions.

From Inspiration to Transformation (The Creation of Guided Imagery and Music, and *Invited by Music)*. 2008. Prod. Eric Bonny and Marilyn F. Clark. Bonny Institute.

Hofmann's Potion. 2002. Dir. Connie Littlefield. Prod. Kent Martin. Atlantic Studio. Film Board of Canada. www.youtube.com/watch?v=4uxvwiwY2OU.

LSD: Documentary on Psychedelic Drugs. 2009. Prod. Caragol Wells. Explorer Series. National Geographic Television. www.youtube.com/watch?v=3aZre1Liboo.

Manna–Psilocybin Mushroom Inspired Documentary. 2003. Prod. and dir. Simon G. Powell. Eco-Shamanic Media. www.youtube.com/watch?v=_xfe7g-3Xuk.

Neurons to Nirvana: Understanding Psychedelic Medicines. 2013. Dir. Oliver Hockenhull. Mangu TV.

Neurons to Nirvana: The Great Medicines. 2014. Dir. Oliver Hockenhull. Moksha Media. www.thegreatmedicines.com.

A New Understanding: The Science of Psilocybin. 2014. Dir. Roslyn Dauber. Prod. Robert Barnhart.

Psychedelic Mysticism: The Good Friday Experiment and Beyond. 2015. Dir. Susan Gervasi. Lazy G Films. www.lazygfilms.net.

Science and Sacraments: Psychedelic Research and Mystical Experiences. 2012. Betsy Gordon Foundation. Prod. Elgin Productions. Psychoactive Substances Research Collection, Purdue University Libraries Archives. www.ScienceandSacraments.com.

A HOPKINS PLAYLIST FOR PSILOCYBIN STUDIES (2008 VERSION)

States of Consciousness Research

WILLIAM A. RICHARDS AND
BRIAN D. RICHARDS

SEQUENCE: COMPOSER, SOURCE OF RECORDING, SELECTION, TIME

Antonio Vivaldi. *Guitar Concerti.* Los Romeros, Iona Brown, Academy of St. Martin in the Fields. Philips 412–624–2
Andante, Concerto RV532 in G Major for 2 guitars, strings, and continuo, 3:30
Largo, Concerto RV93 in D Major for guitar, strings, and continuo, 3:53
Largo, Concerto RV356 in A Minor, 2:20

Paul Horn. *Inside the Taj Mahal.* Kuckuck 11062–2
"Mumtaz Mahal," 3:21
"Shah Jahan," 5:36

Ron Korb. *Flute Traveller: A Musical Journey Across Five Continents.* Oasis Productions, SOCAN NHCD 205
"Alto Flute," 2:16

Russill Paul. *PM Yoga Chants Gaiam.* Relaxation 3142. CD included with the book *The Yoga of Sound.* Novato, Calif.: New World Library, 2004
"By the Stream," 10:54
"Om Namah Shivaya," 2:27

Edward Elgar. *Enigma Variations.* Leonard Bernstein. BBC Symphony. The Artist's Album. DGG 457 691–2
No. 9, "Nimrod," 6:08

Morten Lauridsen. *A Robert Shaw Christmas: Angels On High.* Robert Shaw. Shaw Chamber Singers. Telarc20 CD-80461
"O Magnum Mysterium," 6:13

Russian Orthodox Chant. *Sacred Treasures III, Hearts of Space.* St. Petersburg Chamber Choir, 025041111423
"Alleluia, Behold the Bridegroom," 5:29

Henryk Górecki. *Symphony 3, Op. 36.* Dawn Upshaw. David Zinman. London Sinfonietta. Elektra Nonesuch 9 79282-2
Lento–Sostenuto Tranquillo ma Cantabile, 26:25

Johannes Brahms. *Ein Deutsches Requiem, Op. 45.* Herbert Blomstedt, San Francisco Symphony and Chorus. London 443 771-2
"Selig sind die, da Leid tragen," 10:36
"Denn alles Fleish, es ist wie Gras," 14:33

Johannes Brahms. *Symphony 2 in D Major, Op. 73.* Leonard Bernstein. New York Philharmonic. Sony. SMK 61829
Adagio non Troppo, 10:08

Johannes Brahms. *Ein Deutches Requiem, Op. 45.* Herbert Blomstedt. San Francisco Symphony and Chorus. London 443 771-2
"Wie lieblich sind Deine Wohnungen," 5:34

J. S. Bach. *Mass in B Minor.* Robert Shaw. Atlanta Symphony and Chamber Chorus. Telarc CD-80233
Kyrie I, 10:21
Kyrie II, 4:24

Samuel Barber. *String Quartet, Op. 11.* Leonard Bernstein. New York Philharmonic. Sony SMK 63088
Adagio for Strings, 9:54

Antonio Vivaldi. *Gloria in D Major, R589.* Robert Shaw. Atlanta Symphony and Chamber Chorus. Telarc CD-80194
"Gloria in Excelsis," 2:22
"Et in terra pax," 5:58

J. S. Bach. *Bach Stokowski.* Leopold Stokowski. EMI CDM 7243 5 66385 2 5
"Komm süsser Tod," BMV 478, 5:51

W. A. Mozart. *Vesperae solennes de confessore, K/KV339.* Kiri Te Kanawa. Sir Colin Davis. London Symphony and Chorus. Philips 412 873-2
"Laudate Dominum," 5:11

Johannes Brahms. *Concerto for Violin and Orchestra in D Major, Op. 77.* Jascha Heifetz. Fritz Reiner. Chicago Symphony. HMG 09026- 61742-2
Adagio, 8:12

Henryk Górecki. *Symphony 3, Op. 36.* Dawn Upshaw. David Zinman. London Sinfonietta. Elektra Nonesuch 9 79282-2
Lento e Largo–Tranquillissimo, 9:22

Edward Elgar. *Serenade for String Orchestra, Op. 20.* Mark Elder. Hallé Symphony. CDHLL 7501
Larghetto, 6:29

Gabriel Fauré. *Requiem, Op. 48.* Choir of St. John's College. Cambridge. George Guest. London 436 486–2
"In Paradisum," 3:41

W. A. Mozart, *Clarinet Concerto in A Major, KV 622.* Jacques Lancelot. Jean-François Paillard. Orchestra de Chambre Jean-François Paillard. Erato 2292–45978–2
Adagio, 7:04

Arvo Pärt. *Sanctuary.* Richard Studt. Bournemouth Sinfonietta. Virgin Classics. CSC 7243 5 45314 2 2
"Cantus in Memory of Benjamin Britten," 6:10

Bohuslav Matéj Cernohorsky. *Cernohorsky Religious Works.* Czech Madrigal Singers. Frantisek Xaver Thuri. Gioia Della Musica. Supraphon 11 1598–2 931
"Quare Domine, iraceris–Memento Abraham," 8:58

Ludwig van Beethoven. *Piano Concerto 5 (Emperor), Op. 73.* Leon Fleisher. George Szell. Cleveland Orchestra. Sony SBK 46549
Adagio un Poco Moto, 8:25

Charles Gounod. *St. Cecelia Mass.* Barbara Hendricks. Georges Prêtre. French Radio New Philharmonic. EMI, CDC 7 47094 2
Sanctus, 5:18
Benedictus, 3:16

Russill Paul. *The Yoga of Sound, Shakti Yoga.* Relaxation, CD 3133
"Om Namah Shivaya," 17:35

Richard Wagner. *Tristan and Isolde.* Jesús López-Cobos. Cincinnati Symphony. Telarc CD-80379
Prelude and Liebestod, 17:24

W. A. Mozart. *Grosse Messe C-Moll.* Leonard Bernstein. Chor und Symphonieorchester des Bayerischen Rundfunks. Deutsche Grammaphon 431 791–2
"Ave Verum Corpus," KV618 3:56

Gustav Mahler. *Symphony 5.* Lorin Maazel. Vienna Philharmonic. Sony SBK 89850
Adagietto, Sehr Langsam, 10:33

Alan Hovhaness. *Symphony 2, Op. 132: Mysterious Mountain.* Gerard Schwarz. Royal Liverpool Philharmonic. Telarc 80604
Andante con Moto, 7:42

Joseph Canteloube. *Songs of the Auvergne.* Dawn Upshaw. Kent Nagano. Orchestre de l'Opèra National de Lyon. Erato 0630–17577–2

"Bailèro," 5:36
"Perl'èfon," 3:09

Richard Strauss. *Death and Transfiguration*. André Previn. Vienna Philharmonic.
    Telarc CD-80167
Moderato, 2:20
Tranquillo, 6:03

Russill Paul. *The Yoga of Sound, Nada Yoga*. Relaxation CD 3133
"Evening Shadows Fall," 23:29

J. S. Bach. *Bach Stokowski*. Leopold Stokowski. CDM 7243 5 66385 2 5
Passacaglia and Fugue in C Minor, BMV 582, 14:51

Enya. *Watermark*. Reprise 9 26774-2
"Storms in Africa II," 2:59

Ladysmith Black Mambazo. *Shaka Zulu*. Warner Brothers Collection. Rhino/
    WEA 081227998622
"King of Kings," 4:07

Adiemus. *Pure Moods*. Virgin 724384218621
"Adiemus," 3:59

John Lennon. *The John Lennon Collection*. Abbey Road Capitol 077774644624
"Here Comes the Sun," 3:03

Gipsy Kings. *Mosaique*. Nonsuch 075596089227
"Caminando Por la Calle," 4:22

Mercedes Sosa. Polygram International, Serie Millennium, 042283231429
"Gracias a La Vida," 4:22

Leontyne Price. *The Essential Leontyne Price: Spirituals, Hymns, and Sacred Songs*.
    RCA 090266815722
"Swing Low, Sweet Chariot," 3:24

Louis Armstrong. *What A Wonderful World*. Intercontinental 600 607707405826
"What a Wonderful World," 2:21

NAME INDEX

SUBJECT INDEX

mushroom stone, 82

music, 5, 24, 46, 59, 189–190; body as instrument, 62; choice of, 189–190; Tibetan, 158; unity with, 66–67

mystical consciousness, xxi, 10–11; as delusion or defense mechanism, 45

mysticism: Eastern and Western, 169; study of, 13, 58–59

mysticomimetics, 19

myth, meaning of, 92–93, 212

Nada Brahma, 155

namaste, 57

nameless, the, 42

narcotic addiction, treatment of, xxvii, 80–81, 116–117, 123, 140, 186

Narcotics Anonymous, 125

Nataraja, 46–47

Native American Church, 20, 177

natural childbirth, 12

nature: communion with, 12, 19, 44, 70, intelligence in, 162–164

nausea, 111–112

navigation, principles of, 9

near-death experiences, 136

Negaunee, MI, 199

neo-orthodox theology, 31

Neo-Platonism, 42, 45–46

nervous system, 14, 18, 22, 72, 161, 163

neuroimaging, 141, 146–147

neuroscience, xxviii, 14, 146–147

New Jerusalem, 89

New Mexico, 2005 appeals court ruling, 192

New Testament, 13, 85, 94, 170, 172

New York University, 7, 47, 141, 148

niacin, 31

Nicene Creed, 175

nicotine addiction: attitudes towards, 203; treatment of, 140–141, 150

nicotinic acid, 31

nightmares, 187

nirvana, 10

nitrous oxide, 26, 120

nobility, 15

noetic quality, 32, 39, 65–66, 84, 95, 114

non-drug facilitators of alternate states, 12

non-dual awareness, 42

nonmystical forms of psychedelic experience, 15–16

nonrational experience, 40, 54

norm, deviation from, 21

normality, 21, 70, 185

nothingness, 42

numinous, 42

objectivity and reality, 39

obsessive-compulsive disorder, 122

occult phenomena, 10

ocean, of Brahman, 65

oceanic feeling, 39

Old Testament, 42, 84–85, 91, 172

ololiuqui, 201

"Omega Point," 51

omniscience, 63

openness,16, 55, 114, 131–132, 136, 148, 186, 198

opera metaphor, 92

original blessing, 171

original sin, 171

Orthodox Christianity, 44

Overeaters Anonymous, 125

oxycontin, 150

oxygen, in brain, 12, 15

pain, 104, 148; changed perception of, 47, 110, 135

painting, abstract, 24

palliative care, possible future use of entheogens in, 47

panentheism, 45

panic, 16, 60, 95, 118

panpsychism, 47

marketing of, xix; metabolism of, 14–15; in palliative care, 47; reports of cancer patients, 61–65; synthesis of, xix, 20; in treatment of alcohol addiction, 140–141; in treatment of cocaine addiction, 150; in treatment of depression, 141; in treatment of nicotine addiction, 140; in treatment of obsessive-compulsive disorder, 149

psyche, non-use of term, 22

psychedelic: origin of term, xx; definition, xxix

psychedelic experience: nonmystical forms, 15–16; problems in definition, 19–20; varieties of, xxvii, 16

psychedelic research: author's involvement in, xx–xxii, xxvii; dormant period, 3–4; early history of, xix, 3

psychedelic therapy, 115, 139–143

psychedelics: estimated usage, 7; as medicine, 19; as skeleton keys, 23

psychiatry, biological, 96

psychodelytic therapy, 115

psychodynamic experiences, 16, 104–106

psychodysleptics, 19

psychointegrators, 19

psychology, xxviii

psychology of religion, xxviii, 78

psycholytics, 19

psycholytic therapy, 115

psychonauts, 146

psychosis, 106–108; in early research, xix; screening consideration, 184–185

psychosomatic distress, 108–111, 132

psychotherapy: with alcoholics, 117–118; with cancer patients, 47–48, 61–64, 99–102, 104–106, 108–111; dissolving obstacles, 56, 144; existential/transpersonal, xxviii; with narcotic addicts, 80, 116–117

psychotomimetics, 19

Psychotria veridis, 162

Ptolemaic astronomy, 204–206

pure consciousness event (PCE), 10

"Pure Land," the, xxii, 42, 211

purgation, 34

purgatory, 51, 127

purity, of substances, xxix, 5, 23, 159, 181

Quakerism, 44

rage, 88

range, of alternative states, 23

real relationship, 145

reality, 73, 128, 153–154, 204; of mystical states, xxi–xxii, 33, 39; ultimate, 10–11, 26, 42, 50, 65

reason, 36, 40

rebirth, 64; psychological, 78

reconciliation, 101, 203

recreational use of psychedelics, xxviii, 87, 185

redemption, 54

reductionism, 13–14

regression, 16, 33, 40

reincarnation, 49, 53, 118, 135–136

relationship, personal, with God, 44, 46, 52

relevance, of God concepts, 41

reliability, 12

religion: definition of, 28; dissatisfaction with institutional forms, 28; place of experience within, 26–28

religious professionals, studies with, xxvii

reparenting, 142

resistance, 152, 197

respect, 95

resurrection, 15, 94

retreat centers, entheogens in, 178, 209

revelation, 15, 172; continuing occurrence of, 172–173